THE
Glow
Up

JOURNAL

Everything You Need to Set Goals,
Create Inspo—*and Make It Happen!*

Danielle Richardson, OD

ADAMS MEDIA
NEW YORK LONDON TORONTO SYDNEY NEW DELHI

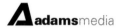

Adams Media
An Imprint of Simon & Schuster, Inc.
100 Technology Center Drive
Stoughton, Massachusetts 02072

First Adams Media hardcover edition May 2023

ADAMS MEDIA and colophon are trademarks of Simon & Schuster.

For information about special discounts for bulk purchases, please contact Simon & Schuster Special Sales at 1-866-506-1949 or business@simonandschuster.com.

The Simon & Schuster Speakers Bureau can bring authors to your live event. For more information or to book an event contact the Simon & Schuster Speakers Bureau at 1-866-248-3049 or visit our website at www.simonspeakers.com.

Interior design by Colleen Cunningham
Interior layout by Colleen Cunningham and Kellie Emery
Interior illustrations by Priscilla Yuen

Manufactured in China

10 9 8 7 6 5 4 3 2 1

ISBN 978-1-5072-2039-9

Contents

Introduction

It's time for the ultimate glow up! Although many people might think of glowing up as having the trendiest clothes, flawless makeup, or tons of *Insta* followers, it's actually about becoming your best and baddest self. It comes from making conscious choices and being an active creator of your reality. In other words, you are the main character of your life, not some supporting role, and a glow up is all about owning that fact. It means manifesting real joy every day—because you are achieving your goals and taking steps toward your happiest, most authentic self.

In *The Glow Up Journal*, you'll plan out your own glow up journey and find all the tools you'll need along the way. You'll focus on bringing that main character energy to each part of your life to make sure that you're truly doing the things that are right for you and what *you* want. In Part 1, you'll take a look at where you're at now and where you want to be. You'll:

- Create schedules and routines for getting things done, like a plan for adapting to whatever changes come your way.
- Figure out the best ways to care for your body, like playing a little exercise bingo.
- Find your unique self-care vibes, like learning to say yes to that much-needed "Me Time."
- See your best life as reality, like creating your own vision board.
- And, of course, customize your baddest self, like creating your personal style.

You'll use fifty journaling prompts to have fun getting to the best version of you. Each chapter in Part 1 ends with a goal-setting practice, so you can keep track of what you've learned and how you want to use that info in your glow up journey.

Then in Part 2, you'll stay on course with tracking pages that bring all the glow up goals you created throughout Part 1 together in one place. Each week, write down what you are working on in each part of your glow up, how often you are committing to working on those goals, and what you will do to stay motivated along the way. And if you slip up (hey, it happens!), this part will also help you get right back into your amazing glow up.

The Glow Up Journal is your guide to defining your dream life, setting goals for what you want, and manifesting those dreams IRL. Your happiest, healthiest self is waiting to claim the awesome life you deserve. So let's get started!

PART 1

Planning Your Glow Up

CHAPTER 1

Everyday Design:
Routines and Scheduling

The key to a lasting glow up is to have a solid foundation. In Chapter 1, you're going to create just that! Your routines and schedules set the framework for your glowed up life because you can't manifest your best and baddest self if there's chaos under the hood. Glowing up doesn't happen overnight; it happens little by little, building lasting change. So it's time to roll up your sleeves and get to it!

In this chapter, you'll create the perfect schedules and daily routines that will help you glow up. You'll be able to better understand your energy levels and at what times of day you are most productive. You'll also focus on designing your days in ways that feel right for you. This is your life, so you get to make the rules for your glow up!

Take the First Step to You 2.0

Let's kick things off by getting clear about where you are right now. If you've picked up this journal, chances are you're probably not satisfied with where things are at in your life. Instead of feeling stuck, use your current state of mind as a starting point! In this activity, you'll take a quick assessment and use it as the start of creating the 2.0 glowed up version of yourself. No matter what brought you here, just know that you are capable of creating change and manifesting a better life! When you finish *The Glow Up Journal*, come back to this activity and compare where you were when you filled it out to where you are once your journal is all done. By committing to this glow up process, you'll leave feeling empowered, inspired, and more fulfilled in your life!

Journal Activity: FULFILLMENT

Mark your current level of fulfillment in each area of life:

MENTALLY

NOT FULFILLED	WORK IN PROGRESS	ALMOST THERE	FULFILLED

PHYSICALLY

NOT FULFILLED	WORK IN PROGRESS	ALMOST THERE	FULFILLED

EMOTIONALLY

NOT FULFILLED	WORK IN PROGRESS	ALMOST THERE	FULFILLED

SPIRITUALLY

NOT FULFILLED	WORK IN PROGRESS	ALMOST THERE	FULFILLED

Do you lean more toward Not Fulfilled or Fulfilled?

Why do you think you lean that direction?

How would you *like* to feel in these areas of your life?

Channel Main Character Energy

Main Character Energy (n): The vibe you exude when you feel like your best self; a.k.a., the most iconic—the baddest—version of yourself!

Life is a movie, and you aren't the supporting role—you're the main character! The main character is the one whose story line viewers follow and who is most connected to the plot. Even if you don't feel like the main character of your life, you are! No matter your circumstances, you can always *choose* to view them in a way that is beneficial. Today, you're going to choose to view yourself as the main character and get to know your main character energy.

Journal Activity: MAIN CHARACTER ENERGY

For this activity, you're going to brainstorm and create the main character version of yourself. Let your imagination run wild and think of the most fabulous, confident, and amazing version of you! How does the main character version of you show up? (*Think about how you look, smell, feel, etc.*)

At the library?

At the office?

At a party?

At a workout class?

With family?

With friends?

With a romantic partner?

On vacation?

Main Character Inspo
Who has this energy? (*List either IRL or fictional characters you love.*)

Understand Your Energy and Natural Cycles

Just like nature has cycles, so do we! You have more energy during certain times of the day than others. In order to glow up and be your best self, you're going to learn to work *with* your natural energy, not *against* it. Over the next few days, you're going to check in with yourself in this journal, taking some notes about how you feel at different times of the day. Keeping a record will help you learn more about yourself and when you have the most energy—and when you have the least.

Journal Activity: ENERGY TRACKER

Over the next seven days, track the times you wake up and go to bed. Rate your energy levels on a scale of 1–5, with 5 being the most energy and 1 being the least.

	M	T	W	T	F	S	S
Time I Woke Up							
A.M. Energy Level							
Midday Energy Level							
P.M. Energy Level							
Time I Went to Bed							
Overall Energy Level							

What wake-up time felt best?

_____

_____

What bedtime felt best?

_____

_____

Based on the chart, what time of day do you usually have the most energy?

_____

_____

How can you use this info to change how you schedule things during your day?
For example, maybe you leave your biggest tasks for the afternoon when you usually
feel the most energized. Or schedule a quick nap for a certain low-energy time. Be
creative with ways you can create a weekly schedule that works for you!

_____

_____

_____

_____

Make Habits That Support Being Your Best Self

Our habits tell us a lot about ourselves because they are who we are when no one else is watching. If we want a different life, we gotta create new habits!

Who isn't guilty of having a few bad habits? The problem comes when those bad habits get in the way of being your best self; that's when you get stuck. The good news is things don't have to stay that way because you have the power to create new habits! Think about the habits of the best version of yourself—a.k.a., Future You! Does Future You hit the snooze button five (or a hundred) times every morning or wake up early? Does Future You skip workouts or commit to an exercise routine? Let's explore the habits that are keeping you from glowing up and brainstorm healthier habits to swap them with.

Journal Activity: HEALTHY HABITS

Habits are simply actions that you repeat over time, often without even thinking about them. For this activity, you'll identify an unhealthy habit you have in each area of life and come up with a healthy habit that can take its place. For example, swap the habit of ordering out most nights with cooking more during the week. Or replace one hour of your daily social media scroll time with a walk! Then answer these questions:

Which habit do you think will be easiest to replace, and why?

_____

_____

_____

Which habit do you think will be most difficult to replace, and why?

_____

_____

_____

	UNHEALTHY HABIT	HEALTHY HABIT
Time Management		
Physical Health		
Mental Health		
Relationships		
Boundary Setting		
Self-Care		

Glow up pro tip: Remember, baby steps add up to change! Create momentum by starting with the easier habits and work your way up to replacing the more difficult ones. Life is a journey, so just take it one step at a time!

Design Your Ideal Day

You know those perfect, wonderful, magical days we all love? These are ideal days: the days spent doing what makes you happy. These special days are usually few and far between, but you can change that by adding elements of your ideal day into your daily life!

What would the day look like if you spent it exactly like you wanted? Let go of any limitations and think of your favorite days in the past. Who were you with? What did you do? What did you eat? You'll use this as inspo to create your vision for your ideal day!

Journal Activity: YOUR IDEAL DAY

Part 1. Defining the Ideal Day

How do you feel during your ideal day?

Where do you go?

What do you do?

How do you relax?

What do you eat?

Who are you with?

Part 2. Designing Your Ideal Day

Based on the answers you wrote, which activities make up your ideal day?

_____

_____

_____

Part 3. Planning Your Ideal Day

On which days of the week could you add an ideal day activity into your schedule?

A.M.	Afternoon	P.M.
M	M	M
T	T	T
W	W	W
T	T	T
F	F	F
S	S	S
S	S	S

Align Your Routines with Your Glow Up Goals

Daily routines offer structure, which helps us have more good days than bad ones. They keep us in alignment with our glowed up self even on the days when we're not feeling it! What exactly *is* a routine? It's a collection of smaller habits that we do consistently, sometimes even without thinking about them.

In order to glow up, you're going to need some new routines to help you become your best self. When you think of Future You, what type of routines do you have? What morning routine helps you set the tone for the day? What evening routine helps you relax and get ready for a good night's sleep? Let's begin to create a routine that keeps you aligned with the glowed up version of yourself.

Journal Activity: A.M. AND P.M. ROUTINES

Part 1. My Glowed Up Morning and Evening Routines
Think about your ideal daily routines for feeling like your best and baddest self. Use the following spaces as a guide to outline your a.m. and p.m. routines.

A.M.	P.M.
When I First Wake Up:	When I First Get Home:
Before Work/School:	How I'll Unwind:
How I'll Nourish Myself Before the Day:	How I'll Nourish Myself after the Day:
How I'll Motivate Myself for the Day:	How I'll Feel Centered:

Part 2. Updating My Current Routines

How do you want to feel each day?

_____

_____

_____

_____

_____

_____

How can you change your current routines to support your feeling this way? (Use your ideal routine from Part 1 of this activity for ideas.)

_____

_____

_____

_____

_____

_____

_____

Make a Schedule That Actually Works

Juggling multiple things every day creates a never-ending to-do list, and we can feel overwhelmed and like we don't have enough time to get it all done. The reality is, you will never be able to cross off every item on your to-do list in one day. Instead, set yourself up for success by prioritizing what needs to get done and planning out your day with a schedule that is realistic.

Schedules shouldn't only be about things you have to get done for others or as part of your responsibilities, though! You also have to schedule in self-care, like working out, reading a book, or spending quality time with loved ones. It's cliché but true: You can't pour from an empty cup. So make sure you are doing something for yourself each day to refill your energy reserves. Including this self-care in your schedule makes you more likely to follow through. Just as you keep your scheduled commitments to others, you're more likely to keep the commitment to yourself!

Journal Activity: DAILY SCHEDULE

Use this template as a guide. Each morning, map out your day and top priorities. Each evening, reflect on how the day went. You can use this daily Glow Up Schedule template in a separate blank journal, date planner, or favorite planning app!

PRIORITIES

DATE: _____ DAY OF WEEK: _____

TODAY I WANT TO FEEL: _____

What are the top three things I have to do today?

1. _____

2. _____

3. _____

How will I take care of myself today?

○ _____ ○ _____ ○ _____

MY SCHEDULE

A.M.

1.
2.
3.

Afternoon

1.
2.
3.

P.M.

1.
2.
3.

END-OF-DAY REFLECTION

What am I most grateful for today?

What did I do well?

What is important for tomorrow?

Adapt to the Busy Pace of Life

When life gets busy, things move fast! If you want to keep your Glow Up on track, you gotta have flexibility and be able to adapt. We all make plans, but let's face it: Sometimes life has a different idea. All schedules are subject to change. Being too rigid can lead to feeling stressed when things don't go your way. Being flexible allows you to go with the flow of life. When things shift, instead of freaking out, you can use powerful quotes to provide that little kick of inspo to get you through!

Journal Activity: QUOTES TO KEEP YOU ON TRACK

What quotes can inspire you to keep going when something unexpected messes up your plans? (*Use your favorite books or look online if nothing comes to mind right away.*) Write them here. Revisit these quotes when you're feeling overwhelmed or unmotivated and need a boost of inspiration to stay on track.

Quote on Motivation:

Quote on Inspiration:

Quote on Trying Again:

Quote on Having Faith:

Quote on Not Giving Up:

Quote on Manifesting Your Dreams:

Stay On Track with Consistency and Self-Discipline

Self-discipline is the ultimate act of self-love. You will never glow up or achieve any of your goals if you aren't consistent—and you develop consistency through self-discipline! Consistency is showing up each day, and discipline is the ability to show up whether or not you feel like it. The key to developing consistency and discipline is to be honest with yourself. Where are you being inconsistent? How can you be more consistent? What new habits will help you build discipline? In this activity, you'll start with a better understanding of the "why" behind your glow up and use that as inspo to help build consistency and discipline.

Journal Activity: CONSISTENCY AND SELF-DISCIPLINE

Take some time now for honest reflection around your "why" and ways to improve.

Why do I want to glow up?

_____

What motivates me to keep going when things get hard?

_____

How am I inconsistent with my...

Health goals?   Self-care goals?

_____   _____

Success goals?   Self-love goals?

_____   _____

Relationship goals?   Money goals?

_____   _____

How can I be more consistent?

_____

How can I be more disciplined?

_____

Goal Setting
Create Your Weekly Glow Up Schedule

Put everything you've learned in this chapter together for your Glow Up Schedule!
Use this template at the start of each week to make sure you're staying on track.

WEEKLY FOCUS

This week's goals:

○ _____   ○ _____   ○ _____

○ _____   ○ _____   ○ _____

This week's healthy habits:

○ _____   ○ _____   ○ _____

○ _____   ○ _____   ○ _____

This week's inspirational quote:

_____

_____

I'm going to stay on track this week by:

_____

_____

What am I grateful for in this upcoming week?

_____

_____

How will I stay focused on my goals this week?

_____

_____

Fill in each day with priorities and important tasks and deadlines for the week ahead. Also, plan things you'll do for yourself, especially on busy days or during busier weeks!

	Today's Priorities	What I'll Do for Me Today
M		
T		
W		
T		
F		
S		
SUNDAY: REST		

CHAPTER 2

Your Body Is a Temple: Diet and Exercise

t's easy to be mean to our bodies and criticize ourselves. We constantly hear and see ideas of what our bodies "should" look like—just scroll through that *Insta* feed and you'll know what I mean! This makes us feel bad about ourselves when we can't measure up to those unrealistic standards. Instead of being so harsh to yourself, check out another way to look at things.

Your body is a temple for your unique spirit; it should be treated with respect and care. How do you treat your most prized possessions? How do you talk about them and protect them? Why *wouldn't* you care for your body the same way?! Instead of looking at your body as an imperfection that needs to be changed, look at it as your Divine Gift. Your body takes care of you and allows you to move through the world. In this chapter, you'll explore tools and practices for taking care of your amazing temple and giving it the glow up it deserves.

Eliminate Toxins

In today's world, we have nonstop exposure to toxins like heavy metals and chemicals found in everything from plastic bottles to our haircare and skincare products. Over time, these toxins can make us sick. The *good* news is our bodies have a natural detox system! The body is an awesome gift, and it can heal itself in the right conditions. This means we don't have to rely on magic pills or formulas when we are in need of a detox.

Toxins that are harmful can also be nonphysical, like negative self-talk or tension with someone you care about. These toxins need to be kicked out of the body too! When you eliminate physical and nonphysical toxins, you give your body a helping hand in its detox process. Ask yourself, "What do I need to remove from my life to give my body time to cleanse itself?"

Journal Activity: YOUR DETOX

Let's think about some of the toxins you come in contact with on a regular basis.

Physical Toxins: (*found in your food, personal and household products, air, water, and other elements of your environment*)

_____   _____

_____   _____

_____   _____

Nonphysical Toxins: (*emotional toxins like self-criticism, financial toxins like overspending, and spiritual toxins like judgment of yourself and others*)

_____   _____

_____   _____

_____   _____

It's time to kick your body into detoxing gear by getting rid of those toxins! Use the following questions as a guide to design a detox plan that is tailored to your goals.

Your Detox Planning Guide

For how many days will you cut out toxins? (*You can eliminate toxins for any amount of time that feels right for you—three days, seven days, thirty days.*)

Which of the toxins that you come in contact with will you focus on eliminating?

What are nontoxic replacements for these (*e.g., swapping heavy cleaning products for organic ones, replacing social media scrolling with a thirty-minute workout*)?

How do you feel pre-detox?

How do you want to feel post-detox?

Post-Detox Check-In
After completing your detox, how do you feel? How will this detox experience affect your lifestyle moving forward?

Use Movement As Medicine

Our bodies are powerful, intelligent, and have a good memory. They can hold onto emotional energy and physical tension. All of this extra-ness in the body can cause issues like disease if ignored for too long. You've gotta move your body to clear every-thing out! It's true: Studies have found that 150 minutes of moderate-intensity aer-obic exercise per week can keep you healthy and reduce the risk of chronic diseases like high blood pressure and diabetes. That's five thirty-minute workouts, or three fifty-minute ones, per week—totally doable!

In this activity, you're going to explore different movement styles and see how you feel after each one.

Journal Activity: MOVEMENT AS MEDICINE

How do you like to move? Brainstorm your favorite movement practices for the dif-ferent styles (relaxing, high-energy, meditative, stress-relieving). Be creative! Jump-ing, dancing, walking, and yoga all count. Then, try each type of movement and write down how you feel afterward in the spaces to the right.

When would each kind of movement be useful for you? (*What time of day, day of the week, or situation would relaxing versus high-energy movement styles work best for you? When could you benefit from meditative movement?*)

Relaxing movement is best when:

High-energy movement is best when:

Meditative movement is best when:

Stress-relieving movement is best when:

Relaxing Movement:
(e.g., yoga, walking)

○ _____

○ _____

○ _____

How I Feel Afterward:

○ _____

○ _____

○ _____

High-Energy Movement:
(e.g., cycling, HIIT workout)

○ _____

○ _____

○ _____

How I Feel Afterward:

○ _____

○ _____

○ _____

Meditative Movement:
(e.g., Yin Yoga, running)

○ _____

○ _____

○ _____

How I Feel Afterward:

○ _____

○ _____

○ _____

Stress-Relieving Movement:
(e.g., Pilates, stretching)

○ _____

○ _____

○ _____

How I Feel Afterward:

○ _____

○ _____

○ _____

Find Foods That Help You Feel Good

When you eat, you're consuming more than just calories: You are also consuming the energy of the food. Whether you eat natural plant-based foods or delicious but processed chips, the energy of the food becomes a part of you. Food can be helpful to our health, and it can also be harmful. Sometimes when we aren't feeling good, it's because we are eating too many unhealthy foods. Your diet should be about 80 percent things that are good for you and 20 percent indulgences you love. If you love some foods that are good for you, so much the better! Think about your current diet and see how much of what you eat is helpful and how much is harmful.

Journal Activity: HEALTHY VERSUS HARMFUL FOODS

Brainstorm and categorize your current diet and favorite foods. Which foods are healthy and helpful? Which are not-so-healthy indulgences?

Healthy + Helpful Foods	Not-So-Healthy Indulgences

Which healthy foods could you eat more of each week?

○ _____   ○ _____
○ _____   ○ _____
○ _____   ○ _____
○ _____   ○ _____
○ _____   ○ _____
○ _____   ○ _____
○ _____   ○ _____
○ _____   ○ _____

Which indulgences are nonnegotiable (a.k.a., you *have* to have at least once a week)?

○ _____   ○ _____
○ _____   ○ _____
○ _____   ○ _____

What is the healthy version of your nonnegotiable indulgences? Do some research and find a way to turn your favorite guilty pleasures into a healthy treat. This will give you flexibility to enjoy your indulgence both the regular way and in a healthier way!

➡ _____
➡ _____
➡ _____
➡ _____
➡ _____
➡ _____

Figure Out Your Ideal Eating Style

There are a ton of different "styles" of eating out there. Some say the newest way is the best, but that may not be true for you. Intuitively, you know what's best for your body!

Read about the eating styles here and circle the one(s) that most interest you. Then look up recipes online and commit to making one of those recipes this week. (Just be sure to talk to your doctor before making a dietary change, to make certain that the style will support your body's needs and not interfere with any medications.)

Journal Activity: IDEAL EATING STYLE

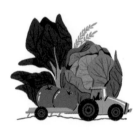 **Whole Foods, Plant-Based:** A whole foods, plant-based diet emphasizes whole, minimally processed foods and limits animal products and food from artificial sources (like added sugars, white flour, and processed oils). When possible, an emphasis is also placed on the quality of food—locally grown, organic, sustainably farmed, wild-caught, seasonal, no GMOs.

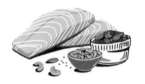 **Paleo:** The paleo diet is meant to mimic the diet of our hunter-gatherer ancestors during the Paleolithic era (about 2.5 million to 10,000 years ago) and emphasizes whole foods, protein, fruits and vegetables, and nuts and seeds.

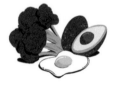 **Keto:** Also known as the ketogenic diet, keto is a low-carb, high-fat diet that focuses on lowering blood sugar and insulin levels.

 Vegan: A vegan diet omits all animal products, from meat to foods like honey, milk, and eggs.

Which eating style would you like to incorporate into your diet? What made it stand out to you as the style your glowed up self would eat?

_____

_____

What will be the easiest part of incorporating this eating style?

_____

_____

What will be the most challenging part of incorporating this eating style?

_____

_____

What recipe did you find for this style that you want to try?

_____

What are the recipe ingredients?

○ _____   ○ _____   ○ _____

○ _____   ○ _____   ○ _____

○ _____   ○ _____   ○ _____

Which foods would make good snacks and easy grab-and-go options for this eating style?

○ _____   ○ _____

○ _____   ○ _____

Find Your Superstar Supplements

Our bodies need vitamins and minerals that we often can't get just from our modern diets alone. This is where nutritional supplements come in! Supplements help us support our bodies and keep things in balance (or get them into balance). You know how a superstar requires a makeup artist, fashion stylist, PR team, and more to be their best on the red carpet? Well, think of yourself as the star and supplements as your support team for being *your* best self!

How do you know what supplements to take? Your primary care physician can test your body's nutrient levels or you can consider at-home testing to find out which vitamins and minerals you may need more of. Keep in mind that supplements aren't FDA-regulated. Be sure to get supplements from manufacturers you trust who use clean ingredients. Always stop taking supplements if you have a reaction and contact your physician.

How do you know if a supplement works? Not all supplements are created equal. Look up brands that create supplements in each of the different categories you are interested in. Look for brands that have full ingredient lists and have data about effectiveness on their websites. Always buy supplements from health food stores because their product quality is better than in supplements found in commercial grocery stores. If you buy supplements online, make sure you go through the company website or another trusted source.

Journal Activity: SUPPLEMENTS

Where could supplements give you a boost? Circle the areas you are interested in giving a little help from a supplement:

ENERGY   FOCUS   RELAXATION

STRESS RELIEF   NUTRITION

Now, take some time to look into different recommended supplements for the things you circled. Use the following list to jump-start your research (add to the list as you learn more!) and be sure to check in with your doctor before starting a supplement.

Energy

- O B Vitamins
- O Coenzyme Q10 (CoQ10)
- O Iron
- O _____

Focus

- O L-Theanine
- O Omega 3
- O Green Tea
- O _____

Relaxation

- O Magnesium
- O Ashwagandha
- O Chamomile
- O _____

Stress Relief

- O Rhodiola
- O Lemon Balm
- O Ashwagandha
- O _____

Nutrition

- O Multivitamin
- O Daily Greens Supplement
- O _____

What is one supplement you can add to your health routine?

_____

_____

_____

Where will you buy the supplement?

_____

_____

What time of day will you take it?

_____

_____

What, if any food, do you need to take with it?

_____

_____

How many days per week will you take it?

_____

_____

Mix 'n' Match for Your Best Workout Routine

The secret to a consistent workout plan is to find something you love to do. Your workout routine will naturally go through phases and cycles too, so it's important to have a few options to choose from. There may be times of the month when you have more energy and want to hit a boxing class and other times when you are less energetic and opt for a Yin Yoga class instead. Changing up your workout styles regularly allows you to stay motivated and consistent even as your energy levels change.

Journal Activity: THE BEST WORKOUT ROUTINE FOR YOU

How many different workouts can you complete this month? Try different ones either in person or at home (or both!), and see if you can hit bingo by crossing each workout off once completed!

End-of-Month Check-In

Which workouts were your favorites?

What did you like about them?

Mat Pilates	Treadmill Intervals	Spin	Orange Theory	Kickboxing
TRX or Strap Workout	At-Home Yoga	Boxing	Rowing	HIIT
Booty Focused Workout	Pilates (Reformer or Megaformer)	Free Space for Any Workout	Barre	At-Home Workout
Any Group Class	Boot Camp	Hot Girl Walk	Yin Yoga	Step Aerobics
Hot Yoga	Strength Training	Dance Fitness	Circuit Training	Cycling

How will you incorporate these workouts into your current routine?

Get Your Gut Into Balance

Keeping your gut healthy keeps your whole body healthy. When you eat unhealthy foods, it throws your gut bacteria out of balance. This imbalance can show up in different ways—stomachaches, bloating, acne, headaches, and a foggy brain, to name a few. There are foods and herbs that help rebalance your gut, but you'll have to make lifestyle changes to keep your gut truly happy. (*One note: Be sure to talk to your doctor before making any dietary changes.*)

Keys to a Healthy Gut

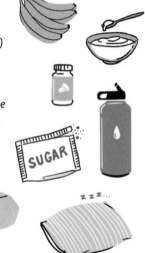

○ Eat foods with fiber (*e.g., bananas, apples, green peas, broccoli, Brussels sprouts, potatoes, black beans, pistachios*)

○ Eat probiotic fermented foods (*e.g., kombucha, kefir, miso, plain probiotic yogurt containing live cultures*)

○ Include probiotic supplements that work for you (*e.g., live probiotic drinks from health food stores, high-quality single strain or multistrain probiotic capsules*)

○ Avoid processed sugars and sweeteners

○ Drink plenty of water

○ Move your body regularly

○ Get plenty of sleep

Journal Activity: GUT HEALTH

How would you rate your current gut health?

○────────○────────○────────○────────○
1: NEEDS A LOT OF WORK   5: FEELS SUPER HEALTHY/NO STOMACH ISSUES

Using Keys to a Healthy Gut as a guide, what are small changes you can make to your lifestyle to improve your gut health?

_____

_____

Craft the Perfect Yoga Routine

Yoga is another awesome way to release energy and tension from the body. More than a workout, yoga combines meditation, self-discipline, and breathing practices to reconnect us with our whole selves. The more yoga you practice, the more it becomes about what you do off your mat: As you connect with your inner self, your outer self starts to change. Yoga teaches the art of living a happy and healthy life!

There are different yoga lineages, but Western yoga is primarily rooted in asana, or the physical postures. Check out the different styles of asana yoga online, consult your doctor, and then practice!

Journal Activity: YOGA EXPLORATION

Pick three yoga styles and follow a short (thirty minutes or less) *YouTube* yoga class in each. Once you've done the classes, journal about how they felt and use this info to craft your own personal yoga routine!

Style of Yoga	How I Felt Afterward	I'll Do This Yoga When...

Hit the Restart Button

You aren't a machine—and you weren't meant to be. Although the goal is consistency, life happens. It's natural to have periods when you're on top of your health and other periods when you're not. The key is to give yourself grace and find your balance. When you fall off track with your wellness glow up goals, the only way to restart your health journey is to show yourself kindness and love. Seek to motivate and inspire yourself, not beat yourself up!

Affirmations are encouraging and empowering statements you can use to remind yourself of the positive possibilities ahead—and that you are capable of achieving them. When you're being hard on yourself, affirmations can be a great pick-me-up. Don't feel guilty about falling off track; it happens! Instead, use affirmations to shift your focus and motivate you to get back in the glow up game.

Journal Activity: SELF-EMPOWERMENT

Create empowering affirmations that you can turn to when you need some inspo to jump back into your health goals (and a reminder of who you are).

Affirmations about Strength: (e.g., "I am capable of anything")

Affirmations about Health: (e.g., "My body is a temple and I love to care for it")

Affirmations about Getting Back in the Game: *(e.g., "I am confident I can become my best self")*

Affirmations about Your Potential: *(e.g., "I am limitless and powerful")*

Affirmations about Staying Positive: *(e.g., "I welcome positivity into my life")*

Goal Setting
Create Your Weekly Food and Movement Plan

Let's put everything you've learned in this chapter together to create your food and movement plan! Use this template each week to make sure you're staying on track.

FOOD PLAN

Healthy foods I'm going to eat more of:

- ○ _____
- ○ _____
- ○ _____

- ○ _____
- ○ _____
- ○ _____

Foods I'm going to eat for my gut health:

- ○ _____
- ○ _____
- ○ _____

- ○ _____
- ○ _____
- ○ _____

MOVEMENT PLAN

How I'll move my body this week:

- ○ _____
- ○ _____
- ○ _____
- ○ _____
- ○ _____
- ○ _____
- ○ _____
- ○ _____

How will you schedule this week's movement? *(Be sure to include rest!)*

M	
T	
W	
T	
F	
S	
S	

Weekly Affirmations
This week's affirmations to support my healthy lifestyle:

CHAPTER 3

Self-Care: Holistic Tools and Practices for Wellness

Your glow up isn't just about the end result; it's also about enjoying the journey to becoming your best and baddest self! While you are doing the glow up work of creating small changes and building new habits, it's important to take care of yourself. It's easy to focus so much on getting to the destination that you neglect your full self along the way, leading to burnout, stress, even health issues. Self-care helps you feel good while on the journey!

Self-care is seen all over social media as face masks and bubble baths—but that's just the surface of self-care. True self-care is about having a holistic view and caring for yourself mentally, physically, emotionally, *and* spiritually. It's about learning what makes you tick and creating practices that help you stay centered and recharge when your energy is low. In this chapter, you'll redefine self-care and create a weekly routine that you can use to support your glow up.

Stop the Stress Sickness

Modern life brings along so much stress! Everyone knows that. But did you know that there are two types of stress? There's positive stress—like excitement before a big game. And there's negative stress—like anxiety or worry. It's healthy to experience both positive and negative stress, but it becomes unhealthy if we have too much negative stress for too long. Negative stress turns on the body's fight-or-flight system. This is good if we're in danger, but bad over time.

Cortisol is your main stress hormone, and too much of it can make you sick. Brain fog, insomnia, and digestive problems are some of the ways too much cortisol (a.k.a., stress) shows up in your life. Over time, too much stress can cause more serious problems like diabetes, high blood pressure, and heart disease.

Good stress management habits now will help you avoid getting sick later! Let's think about the stress you currently experience and how it makes you feel.

Journal Activity: STRESS EVAL

YOU CAN USE POSITIVE/NEGATIVE EMOJIS!

WHAT MAKES YOU FEEL STRESSED?	TYPE OF STRESS

How does stress feel in your body?

How do you feel mentally when you're stressed?

How do you de-stress? What provides stress relief?

Define Your Optimal Health

We've all heard "Health is wealth," but what does it actually mean to be healthy? Just thinking of the word "healthy" brings lots of different opinions to mind. One expert says "this" is healthy while another says "that" is healthy. It can be confusing!

Let's clear things up by defining health on *your* terms. When you define health for yourself, this definition becomes your guiding light. You're able to follow your own intuition about your health and not be confused by all the outside noise.

Journal Activity: OPTIMAL HEALTH

What does it look like to you to have optimal health...

Mentally?

Physically?

Emotionally?

Spiritually?

Reflecting on your answers, create your own definition of "healthy":

Healthy (adj.):

Use Sleep As Self-Care

Sleep is usually left out of the self-care convo, but it shouldn't be! During sleep, your body gets the rest and rejuvenation needed. When you don't get enough sleep, you may feel foggy and/or irritable, and you're more likely to get sick. It's important to create a routine for getting quality sleep.

The goal should be to get between seven and nine hours of sleep every night. Of course, life happens, and it may not always be possible, so just commit to doing your best. For the next week, you'll be mindful of your bedtime and take some notes. These notes will give you clues about what bedtime is best for you and what bedtime routine(s) supports you in getting the best sleep.

Journal Activity: SLEEP TRACKER

Day	Bedtime	Bedtime Routine	Wake Time	How I Felt
M				
T				
W				
T				
F				
S				
S				

Which day did you feel the best?

What was the best bedtime routine for you?

Based on the info collected from your Sleep Tracker, what's your ideal bedtime and your ideal bedtime routine?

Say Yes to "Me Time"

Most people don't have enough time to themselves. We pack our schedules with commitments to others and end up putting ourselves on the back burner. Not anymore! Me Time is your special time for relaxation and rejuvenation. It's a time to be "selfish" in the sense of prioritizing *you*. Me Time is vital for your glow up because it gives you a chance to reconnect with yourself while restoring your energy. When you begin to regularly incorporate Me Time into your lifestyle, you'll notice that you feel happier and more in alignment with yourself!

Journal Activity: ME TIME

Let's figure out what Me Time looks like to you and commit to making it a part of your schedule. Jot brief answers to the following questions.

When are you most excited?

When do you have the most fun?

When are you the most creative?

When do you feel relaxed?

Where can you go to experience these emotions? What types of events or activities leave you feeling excited, creative, relaxed, inspired—or are just plain fun?!

Hot Date Activity

Use your journal answers to create a Me Time date based on how you want to feel (excited, relaxed, creative, etc.) and what helps you feel that way. Describe your date here and schedule it for this weekend, sometime next week, or across multiple days! Your date doesn't have to be an elaborate hours-long affair, but it must be time dedicated to *you*. It should be treated with importance. The primary goal is for you to do an activity IRL, just for yourself. No guilt. No excuses. No procrastination. You'll set a positive tone for yourself by cultivating some self-love!

Practice Some Relationship Self-Care

Relationships are all about boundaries and respect. Boundaries are our limits—a.k.a., what we feel comfortable with versus uncomfortable with. For example, you may be comfortable sharing some personal deets with new friends but draw the line at sharing more intimate info about your love life. You have to respect yourself enough to enforce your boundaries and respect the boundaries of your friends, family, and romantic partner(s) too. This activity will require you to be honest with yourself about your current relationships so that you can figure out what boundaries are needed and where. Creating awareness of these not-so-comfortable truths is the first step of being able to have boundaries that work for you.

Journal Activity: RELATIONSHIP BOUNDARIES

Where are you draining yourself in relationships?

Where do you feel like you are giving too much?

Which relationships feel one-sided?

Which relationships make you feel unappreciated?

Now that you've answered the tough questions, let's think about some ways you can reframe your answers into boundaries to help you get what you need. One example has already been provided.

Issue in Relationship	Boundary Needed	How I Can Set This Boundary
[Person's name] asks me for too many favors.	No more giving favors (unless I really want to and can without it being draining).	"I love being able to help you out when I can, but I'm not able to do this favor."

Take Healing Into Your Own Hands

Your body is constantly giving you info about what it needs, like feeling thirsty when you need water or feeling tired when you need sleep. You are your own best healer because you can sense these things first.

Your intuition is the gift that lets you connect with this kind of inner knowing. And you can strengthen your intuition by slowing down and learning to actively listen to your body. During this activity, you'll strengthen your connection to your body. Get excited, because we're going to get a little "Woo Woo" here!

Journal Activity: BODY SCAN MEDITATION

First, follow these steps to get ready:

1. Dim the lights to create a relaxing ambiance.
2. Turn on relaxing instrumental music. Limit distractions by putting your phone on Do Not Disturb, making sure you are in a quiet space, etc.
3. Create a comfortable area and lie down.

Now, follow these steps to do a body scan meditation:

1. Place one hand over your heart and one on your belly.
2. Close your eyes and just breathe for a moment. Feel your chest rise from your heartbeat and your belly rise from your breath.
3. With your eyes still closed, check in with how you're feeling in each area of the body. Start at the head and scan down to your toes.

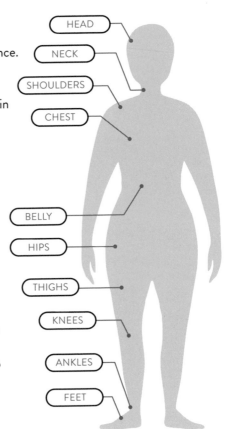

HEAD
NECK
SHOULDERS
CHEST
BELLY
HIPS
THIGHS
KNEES
ANKLES
FEET

Post-Meditation Reflection

Did any part of your body hurt?

_____

_____

Did any part of your body feel tense? Or like it held a lot of pressure?

_____

_____

Did your body give you any messages or did any specific thoughts come up?

_____

_____

How do you feel post–body scan?

_____

_____

Repeat this meditation as often as you'd like!

Care For Yourself Holistically

Self-care means taking care of your full self. It goes deeper than the surface-level care you might immediately think of, like getting your hair done or resting when you feel sick. As you start to explore holistic self-care in this activity, I want you to go beyond the first thoughts that come to mind. Set a timer for five minutes and think about all the self-care activities and practices you've ever heard of—from those over-the-top celebrity self-care practices to simple things that help you take care of your mind, emotions, body, and soul right at home.

Journal Activity: HOLISTIC SELF-CARE

Self-Care for Your Mind. Mental self-care includes activities and tools that help you declutter your mind and reduce mental tension:

_____

_____

Self-Care for Your Body. Physical self-care includes activities and tools that help improve your physical health and well-being:

_____

_____

Self-Care for Your Emotions. Emotional self-care includes activities and tools that help you process and release emotional tension in a healthy way:

_____

_____

Self-Care for Your Soul. Spiritual self-care includes activities and tools that help you align and connect with your Higher Self and Higher Power:

_____

_____

Design a Self-Care Toolbox

There are a lot of self-care practices and tools, but you will be drawn to certain ones. Now that you've brainstormed self-care for each category of mind, body, emotions, and soul, you're going to edit these ideas down into a personalized self-care toolbox. Your self-care toolbox should be full of the things that always help you feel better and help you show yourself some love! It's your quick and easy go-to tool kit for nurturing yourself.

Journal Activity: SELF-CARE TOOLBOX

Flip back to the practices and tools you brainstormed in the last activity. What stands out to you in each list as something that would help you take care of yourself? Write these tools in your personal toolbox.

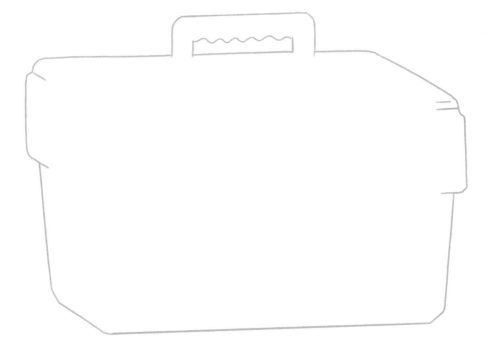

Come back to this toolbox whenever you're in need of a little TLC!

Make Self-Care a Habit

It's debated if new habits take three weeks or sixty-six days to sink in, but we aren't getting that specific here! No matter how long it takes to make a habit, it is always a result of consistently doing a behavior.

It can be hard to create new habits and stick to them. For your glow up, you're going to make it easier by focusing on *trying*. You're going to make the effort each week to incorporate more self-care activities into your routine and track your progress to encourage these activities to become new habits. Start with the goal of committing to self-care activities three times per week, and use the following monthly scheduler to make your schedule and to keep track of how things go.

Journal Activity: SELF-CARE HABITS

Write in three self-care activities for each week of the month. Start with a main self-care goal you have for the week, to help guide your activities. Reuse the weekly template to fill in the activities for each week. Look at a calendar to plan your self-care around any travel, big projects, or celebrations. Planning ahead is the key to success!

WEEK OF	M	T	W
○ COMPLETED			
○ COMPLETED			
○ COMPLETED			
○ COMPLETED			

Weekly Self-Care Activity Goal for
Week 1:

Weekly Self-Care Activity Goal for
Week 3:

Weekly Self-Care Activity Goal for
Week 2:

Weekly Self-Care Activity Goal for
Week 4:

T	F	S	S

Goal Setting
Create Your Self-Care Routines

Let's put everything you've learned in this chapter together to create your self-care routines! When thinking of your self-care routine, you want to think about it in cycles. Don't put pressure on yourself to have the same self-care routine 365 days a year. Just as the seasons change, so should your routines! You need different things at different times of the year—like more moisturizer in winter and more hydration in summer. Let's follow the cues of nature and think about seasonal self-care as you create a holistic routine that feels good.

SEASONAL SELF-CARE CHECKLIST

Spring Self-Care:

○ _____
○ _____
○ _____
○ _____
○ _____
○ _____

Fall Self-Care:

○ _____
○ _____
○ _____
○ _____
○ _____
○ _____

Summer Self-Care:

○ _____
○ _____
○ _____
○ _____
○ _____
○ _____

Winter Self-Care:

○ _____
○ _____
○ _____
○ _____
○ _____
○ _____

Now, let's focus on the current season and think more specifically about self-care activities that can be done on a weekly basis in each of the following categories.

Current Season:

Self-Care for Your Mind:

○ _____

○ _____

○ _____

○ _____

Self-Care for Your Body:

○ _____

○ _____

○ _____

○ _____

Self-Care for Your Emotions:

○ _____

○ _____

○ _____

○ _____

Self-Care for Your Soul:

○ _____

○ _____

○ _____

○ _____

CHAPTER 4

See It to Believe It: Visualizing and Preparing for Your Dream Life

I f you can see it, you can be it! Your thoughts and imagination are a powerful force that give you the ability to create your dream glowed up life. The problem is that most of us are not using this power wisely. Instead, we are often complaining about what's going wrong (hey, it's easy to focus on the bad and forget the good!) and feeling helpless and stuck instead of feeling empowered to make changes to get what we want.

In this chapter, you're going to get unstuck from your current reality. It's time to let go of limiting beliefs and start to dream *big*. What would your life look like if there were no limits? What would you do if you couldn't fail? The activities here are going to help you expand your mindset and create a road map for your dream life.

Get Creating (Instead of Complaining!)

When we want to change something in our life, it's often because we're over it...our job, our money problems, our love life, and just about everything! And when we're in this type of funk or rut, we tend to complain—*a lot*. But complaining is an energy drain. It sucks the life out of you. What if you shifted your energy from complaining to creating? What if, instead of thinking about everything that could go *wrong*, you could focus on what could go *right*? What if you let go of limiting beliefs and opened yourself up to limitless possibilities?

You have the power to flip your mindset and create the life of your dreams! For this activity, you're going to let go of where things currently are and focus only on the awesome things that are to come.

Journal Activity: YOUR DREAM LIFE

What would your life look like without limits? What choices would you make if you could not fail? Imagine your fully glowed up self in the future and write all about what you see. For this particular glow up vision, center your happiness: What will make you the happiest? The most important part of this activity is that you let yourself imagine a future as big and bright as you possibly can, and put that image down onto the page. Let go of limits and allow yourself to *dream*!

This activity requires a timer. Set it for ten minutes to give yourself ample time to brainstorm answers to these questions. It may feel challenging, but commit to using the full amount of time. Feel free to bounce around between categories or move section by section with bullet points, full sentences, or even drawings. Set your timer and let's go!

Who I Want to Be	What I Want to Do	What I Want to Have

Imagine Your Life As a Movie

Imagination is what separates humans from all of earth's other living creatures. We have the ability to bring our dreams into reality! But we tend to lose this spark as we grow up. We start to become more jaded and "realistic" and limit ourselves to the world we can see in front of us.

Let's rediscover the power of your imagination by creating a movie of your life! If you were writing a movie starring the glowed up you, what would the movie be like? Whatever the mind can see and visualize can happen IRL.

Journal Activity: YOUR GLOWED UP MOVIE

It's time to start manifesting the glowed up life you want by using your imagination to create a vision for Future You.

Where Do You Live?

What Do You Do for Work?

What Do You Do for Fun?

How Are You Dressed?

There are no limits here! Use these questions as a guide and brainstorm the best version of your life at different time periods. Get detailed, so you can really see it playing out like a movie. Ready...action!

My life in one year:

My life in ten years:

My life in five years:

My life in twenty years:

Explore What Success Looks Like for You

We often chase an idea of being successful, but what does that even mean? Society, our families, and the media can give us all kinds of ideas of what success looks like. But sometimes they can have *too* much influence on our definition of success. When this happens, we waste our lives chasing a dream that isn't even ours to begin with. We have to stop and think: Is our idea of success from outside sources, or is it coming from inside ourselves?

To have a true glow up, you need to think of success from a holistic perspective and define it for yourself. It's *your* glow up, after all! In the following journal activity, you're going to expand your thoughts about success to include not just what you can accomplish, but how you feel while accomplishing it. You'll use this new idea of success as the road map to creating your glowed up life!

Journal Activity: GLOW UP SUCCESS ROAD MAP

You can't know where you're going if you don't have a road map! Here, you'll define success for yourself and use this definition as your North Star. Think about how it looks IRL to have success and how it feels to you as well.

DEFINE

Health and Wellness

_____

_____

_____

Career

_____

_____

_____

Finances

_____

_____

_____

Love and Relationships

_____

_____

_____

VISUALIZE

Now, let's create a mental picture! Using your answers as a guide, close your eyes and visualize your successful, glowed up self five years from now. Spend as much time visualizing as you like to really see yourself and your glow up in detail! Then, fill in a couple of action steps you can take this year to get closer to this success in each category:

Health and Wellness

○ _____   ○ _____

Finances

○ _____   ○ _____

Career

○ _____   ○ _____

Love and Relationships

○ _____   ○ _____

Plan Your Dream Career

It's really unfair that right out of school, we're told to choose a career and then stick with it for the next thirty-plus years. This model is outdated and makes people overidentify with their jobs, which makes them miserable in the long run.

In this activity, you'll expand your thinking beyond traditional jobs and instead, think about your career *lifestyle*. You will spend most of your time at work, so you should make sure you're planning to work in a way that makes sense for you and the career lifestyle that you want. You might seek a life of multiple sources of passive income, or maybe you'd prefer a long-term, more involved goal like becoming a judge!

No matter what you choose, keep in mind that you don't have to do things the way they've always been done. This is your friendly reminder to *just do you!*

Journal Activity: DREAM CAREER DESIGN

The following questions will guide you in thinking about career a little differently.

1. What do you want to do for work?
2. What are your professional interests?
3. How much time do you want to spend working?
4. How much time do you want to spend on vacation?
5. Where do you want to work from?
6. How much money do you want to earn?
7. What are jobs that provide your ideal time commitment, money, and location?

Use Social Media for Empowerment

Social media can be a gift…or a curse. Living in the digital age, we see more people in one hour than our grandparents probably saw in their entire lives. This creates hundreds of opportunities every day to compare ourselves with others. Social media on its own is neutral: We are the ones who give it power. Does social media put you in a good energy space and inspire you to become your best self? Or does it put you in a negative energy space and make you feel like you aren't good enough? Social media should be a tool for learning and inspiration on your glow up journey. By choosing to be more selective about who you follow and engage with, you can create a social media experience that brings joy to your life—instead of sadness, frustration, etc.

Journal Activity: SOCIAL MEDIA AUDIT

Let's do a social media "audit" of your current social media experiences. No judgment here—you just want to see where things are at! Answer these questions:

How do you feel after spending time on social media?

Which social media platforms make you feel the best?

Which social media platforms make you feel the worst?

Which social media accounts inspire you, and why?

Which social media accounts make you feel like you're not enough, and why?

What changes can you make to use social media in a way that makes you feel happier and more inspired?

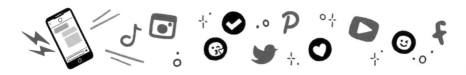

Plan Your Dream Lifestyle

A lot of people think of life in terms of work and/or family. But what if you thought about it from a lifestyle perspective first? Before you go all in on a career or start nurturing a family dynamic, what if you got clear about the lifestyle you want to live to make sure the work and family you choose align with your dream lifestyle?

Your glowed up life is all about being intentional about the decisions you make so you can create your dream reality. While you're on the journey to becoming your best self and creating this dream, you'll be presented with lots of choices and opportunities. If you're clear about the life you want to create, you can make the choices that are best for you much more easily!

Journal Activity: DREAM LIFESTYLE DESIGN

What is most important to you in life?

How do you want to spend your time?

How does your dream lifestyle look and feel?

Describe your dream lifestyle on a daily, weekly, and monthly basis:

Daily: **Weekly:**   **Monthly:**

_____   _____   _____

_____   _____   _____

_____   _____   _____

_____   _____   _____

_____   _____   _____

_____   _____   _____

_____   _____   _____

What are elements of your dream lifestyle that you can implement right now?

○ _____

○ _____

○ _____

○ _____

○ _____

○ _____

○ _____

○ _____

○ _____

Create a Vision Board

You've got to see it to believe it! Being practical and realistic is drilled into us during school, which can make it hard to think any different. But in order to have a glow up, you're going to have to remember that the regular rules don't apply to you! Just because something is the way it is now, doesn't mean it has to be that way forever.

Glowed up baddies see the future before it gets here. How do they do it?! Via vision boards. Vision boards work because of our subconscious mind (a.k.a., the part of our brain that receives info through our senses and works on autopilot). Our subconscious mind is always influencing what we attract into our lives, so you want to feed it inspiration—not negativity. By creating a vision board, you're making a portal that you can look through whenever you need to feel inspired or if you need a little pick-me-up during a tough day. Your vision board will transport you to that version of you that is your best and baddest self! With these images in mind, you'll start to think and act differently in your real life; you'll begin to take inspired action toward your glowed up future, and over time you'll start to realize that your real life resembles your vision board.

Journal Activity: VISION BOARD

You're going to create a vision board for your glowed up life. It's like an art project that is all about you!

How to Create Your Vision Board

Before you start, use the following questions to brainstorm ideas for your board:

What medium will you use for your vision board (e.g., poster board, Pinterest, a blog page)?

What are some key image styles you want to use (*e.g., travel, architecture, happy couples*)?

What are some key words you want to use for your vision board (*e.g., freedom, wealth, love*)?

Now, follow these steps to get creating:

1. Decide on your medium.
2. Find images and words that make you feel good. The key is to *feel* inspired and happy when you look at what's on your board.
3. Arrange all the images and words on your board!

How to Use Your Vision Board

1. **Look at your vision board daily.** Each day, show your subconscious mind your vision board so you can stay inspired and remember what you're creating.
2. **Practice visualization.** Now that you see your vision board with your eyes open, can you still see it with your eyes closed? Practice visualization by finding a quiet space, closing your eyes, and imaging yourself living in the real-life version of your vision board. This can be a challenge at first, so start by practicing for five minutes and then work to visualizing for longer periods.
3. **Add inspo as you go.** Your vision board, just like your life, is a work in progress. Continually add to your board when you feel inspired or think of new ideas for Future You!

Identify Your Strengths (and Weaknesses)

You gotta grow to glow! We are beautifully imperfect humans with our own set of gifts and talents. We also have our own set of flaws. And although we'd rather ignore these flaws, glowed up baddies know that blind spots are bad news.

It's important for you to be aware of yourself—to know your own strengths *and* weaknesses. After all, it's hard to create your dream life when you don't really know who you are. You might be judging yourself because you're trying to do something that isn't in alignment with your natural talents. Your dream life will take work to create, but there will be a sense of ease when you're working within your gifts and not against them. The sooner you can identify your strengths and weaknesses, the better off you'll be. Throughout this journey, remember that your weaknesses are not something to feel bad about. Being aware of your weaknesses allows you to refine them and improve how you show up in the world. So embrace yourself—flaws and all!

Journal Activity: STRENGTH AND WEAKNESS REFRAME

You are going to use one of the best tools to help with self-assessment: the personality test! Personality tests are great ways for you to hear about yourself objectively, but also privately. Complete a personality test using the Myers-Briggs assessment, a numerology calculator, or the Enneagram tests. All of these methods offer free testing online. Once you complete the test, read about your result, and then use what you find out to help you answer the following questions.

What are three of your strengths?

1. _____

2. _____

3. _____

How can you use your strengths?

_____

_____

_____

What are three of your weaknesses?

1. _____

2. _____

3. _____

How can you improve on your weaknesses?

_____

_____

_____

Make Money Your Bestie!

Whether you have too little or more than you know what to do with, *everyone* has a complicated relationship with money. In order to glow up, you'll have to reframe your relationship with money and make it your bestie! Why? Money is an energy just like everything else in the world. And just like with everything else, you can either invite or shut out that energy. You need to build a positive relationship with it in order to manifest it in your life!

Journal Activity: MONEY BFF

How would you rate your current relationship with money?

|—————————+———+———+———+———|———+———+———+———|

WE'RE ENEMIES   WE'RE FRENEMIES   WE'RE BESTIES

What are your early memories of money? What things have your parents said to you about money?

What could be better about your money management (*e.g., using financial apps, creating a monthly budget*)?

How can you increase the money you have?

Goal Setting
Create Your Ideal Life and Lifestyle

By this point in your journaling, you've been able to dream and create goals for yourself. It's time to propel these ideas from your mind into the real world by creating a plan of action. By having a plan in place, you can save yourself time and detours on your journey to that glowed up life. Although you don't always have full control over what happens, you can still be prepared! Let's create a five-year life plan.

FIVE-YEAR LIFE PLAN

What does your life look like in five years?

What steps do you need to take this year to get closer to that vision?

What steps can you take during the next three months to get closer to that vision?

What can you do this week to get closer to that vision?

Fill in the milestone markers on this map to plan out your next five years.

NOW

Milestones:

1. _____
2. _____
3. _____

YEAR
1

Milestones:

1. _____
2. _____
3. _____

YEAR
2

Milestones:

1. _____
2. _____
3. _____

YEAR
3

Milestones:

1. _____
2. _____
3. _____

YEAR
4

Milestones:

1. _____
2. _____
3. _____

YEAR
5

Becoming Your Baddest Self: Beauty and Style

Welcome to your Healthy Baddie Era! Just like Cinderella had a magical glow up before the ball, it's time for you to have a magical glow up into your best and baddest self. What is a healthy baddie? It's someone committed to being the best version of themselves, looking and feeling good while doing so. Becoming your baddest self isn't about appearing trendy; it's about making changes so your inner beauty can shine through!

This chapter will guide you through the final stage of your glow up! Being your baddest self doesn't require a ton of money—just some commitment and maintenance. You have to commit to raising your standards and make the time to maintain those standards. Royal treatment only!

Become the Most Beautiful You

As cliché as it sounds, beauty really does come from within. But how can you access this beauty? How can you become the most beautiful version of yourself? It's really simple but something that can be so difficult to do: You have to be nice to yourself!

We all tend to criticize ourselves and pick apart our flaws instead of celebrating who we are. But if you talked about your bestie the way you talk about yourself, would they still be around? The answer is probably not.

Becoming the most beautiful you starts with self-love and creating a real and loving relationship with the person you see in the mirror. It's time to explore what makes you so worth loving!

Journal Activity: SELF-LOVE PRACTICE

What is your favorite thing about yourself?

_____

_____

_____

_____

What do you love about your personality?

_____

_____

_____

_____

_____

What is your most attractive feature?

What makes you unique?

When do you feel the most beautiful?

Practice Keeping Fresh and Clean Every Day

Becoming your baddest self starts with becoming high maintenance. Hear me out—not high maintenance in the sense of expensive, but maintaining high standards for how you take care of yourself.

Think of the most fab person you know. Chances are their nails are clean, their hair is styled, and there is definitely no B.O. They've invested in good grooming, and you can do the same! Being the baddest version of yourself requires you to be well groomed, and it only requires you take some extra time! This activity will help you identify your grooming goals and plan out a schedule for hitting and maintaining them.

Journal Activity: SELF-MAINTENANCE SCHEDULE

First, what does being well groomed mean to you?

How often do you need "maintenance" in different parts of your grooming routine? This will be different for everyone (e.g., you may need a hair appointment every month or just a quick trim every eight weeks). Think about what you need to feel fresh and clean, and use this chart to help yourself stay on track!

TYPE OF CARE	HOW OFTEN
Body Care: (e.g., shower, body hair removal)	
○	
○	
○	
Hair Care: (e.g., haircut, wash and style)	
○	
○	
○	

TYPE OF CARE	HOW OFTEN
Face Care: (e.g., face mask, facial hair trimming/removal)	
○	
○	
○	
Nail Care: (e.g., manicure, trim)	
○	
○	
○	
Other: (e.g., professional massage)	
○	
○	
○	

Take It Beyond This Journal:
Find some time this weekend to give yourself a little TLC via an at-home spa night. Get some of that grooming maintenance done!

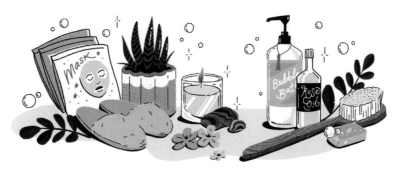

Love the Skin You're In

It's important to love and take care of our skin—not just on the face, but on the whole body. Did you know that the skin is the body's largest organ that eliminates?! That means your skin is constantly getting rid of toxins and things you don't need. It also means your skin can absorb what you put on it. Because of this, you have to be mindful of the products you use. How would you treat a delicate flower? Carefully, right? That's how you should treat your skin: with a lot of care!

Your skin can be sensitive, acne-prone, oily, dry, or a combination of types. Good skin care is about learning your skin type and which products work well for you. You also have to learn which products contain harmful toxins like synthetic fragrances that can be irritating or parabens that can disrupt your hormones.

Journal Activity: THE SKINCARE EDIT

Let's edit your skin and body care products. It's time to get rid of things you don't use, are super toxic, or have expired. When finished, list your favorite products for taking care of your skin. Update this list as you find new favorites to keep a catalog of what works well for you. Don't have any quality products for your face or body? It's time to do a little research and write about what recommendations you find.

Facial Skin Care

Cleansers:

Treatments:

Moisturizers:

Oils:

Body Skin Care

Cleansers:

Treatments:

Moisturizers:

Oils:

Note: Always apply your skincare products from thinnest to thickest, and save oils for the end! Pro tip for body care: Use oil on damp skin after the shower and pat dry.

Look and Feel Expensive (on a Budget!)

Whether or not you're rolling in cash, you can still *look* expensive. Looking expensive is about feeling confident in your appearance. Picking up on someone looking expensive is actually picking up on a person's confidence in knowing they look good! So how do you achieve this look when you don't have a celebrity budget or trust fund? Learn the rules of looking expensive on a budget and how to navigate your expensive tastes.

Journal Activity: YOUR LUXE LOOK

First things first, check out these rules for having champagne taste on a Perrier budget:

1. **Quality over Quantity.** Become discerning and seek out the best thing in your price range. Buy less but choose higher-quality items; explore luxury consignment!
2. **Fit Matters.** If it doesn't fit, don't wear it. Make sure you can walk in those shoes, and don't adjust your clothes in public.
3. **Out with the Old.** Get rid of your old, worn-out clothes. Poorly made clothes show signs of wear and tear more easily, so edit your closet to remove those items. Be sure to donate your gently used clothes.
4. **Timeless over Trendy.** When you have a limited budget, always invest in timeless pieces you'll actually wear over trendy one-offs. Focus on wardrobe staples, choosing the items you will wear regularly. Think shoes, bags, and coats!

Creating Your Luxe Look

Use these questions to create a blueprint for your luxe look! Come back to these answers as you update your wardrobe or before you go shopping.

What does expensive look like to you?

What does expensive feel like to you?

What do you already own that makes you feel expensive?

Develop Your Signature Scent

We all know someone who smells soooo good! What is their secret? They have a signature scent, a.k.a., a customized routine of layering certain fragrances. You can do this too! The cool thing about fragrance is that, thanks to all the different fragrances and layering options out there, it will always smell unique to you.

There are so many opportunities to use fragrance in your life, but you'll want to be smart about it. The ingredient "fragrance" listed on products is a catchall for chemicals, artificial or natural, that give the product scent. Some fragrance chemicals are endocrine disruptors, which wreck your hormones and can cause serious allergies or diseases when used for long periods of time. Each product is different, so always do your research to find brands you trust and scents you love that will keep you safe!

When developing your signature scent, you'll also want to think about how long scents last and what types of scents pair well together. There *is* such a thing as too much fragrance, so try to keep in mind that less is more. And if you have allergies, remember that you can also go fragrance-free!

Journal Activity: FAV SCENT SELECTION

Use this activity to explore scents you love. The categories represent different scents you can include in your routine, but you don't have to use them all. This activity is meant to serve as a guide and give you some ideas!

What types of scents do you like in your...

Shampoo and conditioner?

○ _____

○ _____

○ _____

Detergent?

○ _____

○ _____

○ _____

Body wash?

○ ....

○ ....

○ ....

Body lotion?

○ ....

○ ....

○ ....

Perfume?

○ ....

○ ....

○ ....

Scented oils?

○ ....

○ ....

○ ....

Mist-on fragrances?

○ ....

○ ....

○ ....

Develop Your Signature Style

The best part of life is that we get to reinvent ourselves whenever we want and use our style as a way to communicate that self to the world. But there's a big difference between being trendy and being stylish. Trends will come and go because what goes out of fashion always comes back in fashion and vice versa. Style is more about the clothes you're drawn to and wear over and over again even as the trends come and go. Even if you don't think you were born with style sense, you can always develop a signature style.

Having a strong sense of your style is important in your glow up because you can't be your baddest self if you look to other people to tell you what to wear. You have to be able to listen to your inner baddie and find a style that is unique to you!

Journal Activity: YOUR STYLE

No matter where you're starting out, your style can be cultivated over time. It comes from learning what you think is flattering and what you like to wear. As you get clearer about which styles you gravitate toward, you start to get a better sense of what you like. This activity will help you explore the styles that appeal to you and put your unique spin on them.

Who are your style icons?

How would you describe their style?

How do their clothes fit them? Which silhouettes do they wear?

What color palettes do they wear?

What are your personal style values? Think about what you value and how this translates to your personal style. (*Do you value comfort? Do you value looking professional and being taken seriously? Do you value appearing taller or slimmer?*)

_____

_____

Outfit Pairing Exercise
Use the clothes in your current closet to create outfits inspired by your answers to the previous questions.

Top

+ _____

+ _____

+ _____

+ _____

Bottom

+ _____

+ _____

+ _____

+ _____

Outerwear

+ _____

+ _____

+ _____

+ _____

Shoes and Accessories

+ _____

+ _____

+ _____

+ _____

Understand Your Signature Vibe

Your vibe is the energy you give off. And since it's energetic, it's fluid and will change with your mood and life experiences. Understanding your signature vibe is about knowing yourself and your energy better—because the more comfortable you are with yourself, the more confident you will feel.

Your vibe is unique to you but it can be felt by those around you. Are you normally bubbly and talkative? Or more introspective and reflective? How does your energy shift when you're annoyed? Excited? Anxious? How do you respond to wins? To losses? To change? Understanding how your vibe is impacted by outside influences empowers you with self-awareness. When you know about yourself and how your vibe shifts in different situations, you're able to better regulate your energy and manage how you show up in the world. Becoming self-aware and being able to maintain the vibe you want to bring to your life—no matter what is going on—is a real glow up!

Journal Activity: SELF-ASSESSMENT

Let's explore your vibe. We're going to view it through your eyes and through the eyes of two people closest to you. This will give you some insight into how other people experience your vibe.

Part 1

Ask two people close to you the following question and jot down their answers: What five words would you use to describe me?

Name: _____   Name: _____

1. _____   1. _____

2. _____   2. _____

3. _____   3. _____

4. _____   4. _____

5. _____   5. _____

Part 2
Answer the following questions:

When do you feel your best?

When do you feel the most angry?

When do you feel the most relaxed?

When do you feel the most peaceful?

When do you feel the most annoyed?

When do you feel the most joyful?

Part 3
Using all of the info you've gathered in this activity, how would you define your vibe? Does it change frequently or does it remain consistent? (Remember, this activity is not about judging yourself; it's about understanding yourself better!)

When your vibe feels off, what are things you can do to reset it?

Glamorize Your Life

Glamour isn't just reserved for the weekends or big events. You can bring glamour into your daily life and make even your most mundane tasks a bit more special. This is how you romanticize your life! When you glamorize the small moments, you're able to add more happiness into your life. It can be simple things like making your bed a new way, buying new drinking glasses, or arranging fresh florals in your space every week. Fancy pajamas, silk pillowcases, or a long, leisurely walk to notice beauty can all help you glow up your world via a little glamour.

Journal Activity: YOUR BEST LIFE

For this activity, you're going to brainstorm simple luxuries you can add into your day-to-day. So let's dive in!

What glamour can you add to your morning routine (*e.g., drinking tea from a "fancy" cup, wearing a matching set for your workout, sitting down to eat breakfast without your phone*)?

What glamour can you add to your evening routine (*e.g., lighting a candle while you do your skin care, sleeping in matching pajamas, listening to romantic music*)?

How can you add more glamour to your self-care routine (*e.g., creating a beautiful meditation space, using aromatherapy via essential oil diffuser*)?

Where can you include more leisure time in your schedule (*e.g., going for a walk three times a week, having some relaxation time for an hour after work, creating a new floral arrangement for your space on Sundays*)?

Take It Beyond This Journal
Take a long, leisurely walk and listen to your favorite podcast or playlist. Challenge yourself to stop three times and actually smell the flowers or plants you come across.

Look Out For Your Fab Future Self

It's a blessing to be alive! But we live in a world that glorifies looking younger than you are for as long as humanly possible...which can make the idea of getting older a nightmare. It doesn't have to be, though!

Let's be real. Everyone wants to look good and keep that glow up going regardless of age. The secret to aging gracefully is to take care of yourself *now*, and keep up with that care. Develop good habits in your younger years that will help you be healthy and happy as you get older. Your diet, your movement, and your mindset all play a huge role in how your body ages. And don't forget the world of Botox, laser treatments, anti-aging creams, and more. The spectrum of what you can incorporate into your routine for looking out for Future You is wide, but remember to ignore pressure from the outside world and do what feels good for you!

Things change from decade to decade and from life event to life event. Be sure to prioritize your self-care so you can maintain your essence and experience the gift of aging gracefully!

Journal Activity: FUTURE YOU

It's easy to fear growing old if you have a limited idea of what that actually means. Here, you're going to find inspo from people across several decades of life to prove to yourself that getting older is a gift and can also be fabulous! Use magazines or go online (or both!) to find fab and inspirational people who show just how amazing it can be to mature. What makes someone fabulous to you? Who are the people that fit your definition of fabulous? List the names and ages of your Fab Favs here!

30s Inspo: _____

40s Inspo: _____

50s+ Inspo: _____

Celebrities are always sharing their secrets for aging gracefully. Do some research and see what your Fab Favs have to say about their beauty and style routines as they get older. Is there anything you find that you want to incorporate into your life?

Goal Setting
Create Your Personal Style Guide

Let's put everything you've learned in this chapter together to create your personal style guide! This will serve as a reference you can look to when shopping or refreshing your style. Refer back to your answers for inspo to complete your style guide!

YOUR SIGNATURE STYLE

What fashion styles do you love?

Which silhouettes are most flattering to you?

YOUR STYLE FORMULA

What outfits do you like to wear?

What types of clothes do you need for these outfits?

BEAUTY STYLING

Which hairstyles work for your look?

Which makeup styles and colors looks best on you?

FINISHING TOUCHES

Which accessories suit your style?

What scents do you like to wear?

Glow up pro tip: Don't be afraid to reinvent yourself! You have the power to step into your own New Era at any time, so update this personal style guide as you and your style evolve.

PART 2

Tracking Your Glow Up

Glowing up is an active process. If we want to make our dreams a reality, we have to take the journey to become our best selves and put in the work. How can you do that? It's simple: Create a plan and stick to it! You bring your dream life out of your mind and put it into the real world by tracking your goals along the way.

This part of *The Glow Up Journal* is your personal accountability buddy to help keep you on track of your own ultimate glow up. It offers both support and a reminder of what steps to take and where you're headed. There is a weekly check-in to set the tone for the week and a daily check-in to keep you accountable each day. Have fun filling out the daily templates, and flip back to Part 1 every time you need a refresher on your goals or feel like creating new goals. Remember, there's no one way to glow up, and the best part of glowing up is the process!

Sunday
CHECK-IN

Every Sunday, create dedicated Me Time for you and your glow up by completing this weekly check-in. You'll plan ahead and set the tone for the week while reminding yourself of your glowed up goals!

ROUTINES AND SCHEDULE

I'm going to commit to these goals:

○ _____
○ _____
○ _____
○ _____

I'm working on these healthy habits:

○ _____
○ _____
○ _____
○ _____

I'm going to stay on track by:

○ _____
○ _____
○ _____
○ _____

DIET AND EXERCISE

Healthy foods I'm eating more of:

○ _____
○ _____
○ _____
○ _____

This week's superstar supplement(s):

○ _____
○ _____
○ _____
○ _____

This week's movement goals:

○ _____
○ _____
○ _____
○ _____

BEAUTY AND STYLE

I will look and feel my best by:

○ _____
○ _____
○ _____
○ _____

I will add glamour to my routine by:

○ _____
○ _____
○ _____
○ _____

I will pamper myself by:

○ _____
○ _____
○ _____
○ _____

My big glow up goal for the year is:

This week, I will get closer to my glow up goal by:

I affirm that I *am*:

HOLISTIC TOOLS AND PRACTICES FOR WELLNESS

This week's self-care activities for my:

Mind	Body	Soul
M	M	M
T	T	T
W	W	W
T	T	T
F	F	F
S	S	S
S	S	S

Daily
CHECK-IN

At the end of each day, use the following prompts to check in with yourself and your glow up progress, filling in the chart with your reflections.

MONDAY	TUESDAY	WEDNESDAY

I'm grateful for this:

Glow up wins from today:

Things to remember for tomorrow:

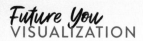

Future You
VISUALIZATION

Now, use your vision board to visualize about your glowed up future for five minutes. Trust that you are becoming your best and baddest self. Your glow up is under way—keep going!

THURSDAY	FRIDAY	SATURDAY	SUNDAY

Sunday
CHECK-IN

Every Sunday, create dedicated Me Time for you and your glow up by completing this weekly check-in. You'll plan ahead and set the tone for the week while reminding yourself of your glowed up goals!

ROUTINES AND SCHEDULE

I'm going to commit to these goals:

- ○ _____
- ○ _____
- ○ _____
- ○ _____

I'm working on these healthy habits:

- ○ _____
- ○ _____
- ○ _____
- ○ _____

I'm going to stay on track by:

- ○ _____
- ○ _____
- ○ _____
- ○ _____

DIET AND EXERCISE

Healthy foods I'm eating more of:

- ○ _____
- ○ _____
- ○ _____
- ○ _____

This week's superstar supplement(s):

- ○ _____
- ○ _____
- ○ _____
- ○ _____

This week's movement goals:

- ○ _____
- ○ _____
- ○ _____
- ○ _____

BEAUTY AND STYLE

I will look and feel my best by:

- ○ _____
- ○ _____
- ○ _____
- ○ _____

I will add glamour to my routine by:

- ○ _____
- ○ _____
- ○ _____
- ○ _____

I will pamper myself by:

- ○ _____
- ○ _____
- ○ _____
- ○ _____

My big glow up goal for the year is:

This week, I will get closer to my glow up goal by:

I affirm that I *am*:

This week's self-care activities for my:

Mind	Body	Soul
M	M	M
T	T	T
W	W	W
T	T	T
F	F	F
S	S	S
S	S	S

Daily
CHECK-IN

At the end of each day, use the following prompts to check in with yourself and your glow up progress, filling in the chart with your reflections.

	MONDAY	TUESDAY	WEDNESDAY
I'm grateful for this:			
Glow up wins from today:			
Things to remember for tomorrow:			

Future You
VISUALIZATION

Now, use your vision board to visualize about your glowed up future for five minutes. Trust that you are becoming your best and baddest self. Your glow up is under way—keep going!

THURSDAY	FRIDAY	SATURDAY	SUNDAY

Sunday
CHECK-IN

Every Sunday, create dedicated Me Time for you and your glow up by completing this weekly check-in. You'll plan ahead and set the tone for the week while reminding yourself of your glowed up goals!

ROUTINES AND SCHEDULE

I'm going to commit to these goals:

○ _____
○ _____
○ _____
○ _____

I'm working on these healthy habits:

○ _____
○ _____
○ _____
○ _____

I'm going to stay on track by:

○ _____
○ _____
○ _____
○ _____

DIET AND EXERCISE

Healthy foods I'm eating more of:

○ _____
○ _____
○ _____
○ _____

This week's superstar supplement(s):

○ _____
○ _____
○ _____
○ _____

This week's movement goals:

○ _____
○ _____
○ _____
○ _____

BEAUTY AND STYLE

I will look and feel my best by:

○ _____
○ _____
○ _____
○ _____

I will add glamour to my routine by:

○ _____
○ _____
○ _____
○ _____

I will pamper myself by:

○ _____
○ _____
○ _____
○ _____

VISUALIZING AND PREPARING FOR YOUR DREAM LIFE

My big glow up goal for the year is:

This week, I will get closer to my glow up goal by:

I affirm that I *am*:

HOLISTIC TOOLS AND PRACTICES FOR WELLNESS

This week's self-care activities for my:

Mind	Body	Soul
M	M	M
T	T	T
W	W	W
T	T	T
F	F	F
S	S	S
S	S	S

Daily
CHECK-IN

At the end of each day, use the following prompts to check in with yourself and your glow up progress, filling in the chart with your reflections.

MONDAY	TUESDAY	WEDNESDAY

I'm grateful for this:

Glow up wins from today:

Things to remember for tomorrow:

Future You
VISUALIZATION

Now, use your vision board to visualize about your glowed up future for five minutes. Trust that you are becoming your best and baddest self. Your glow up is under way—keep going!

THURSDAY	FRIDAY	SATURDAY	SUNDAY

Sunday
CHECK-IN

Every Sunday, create dedicated Me Time for you and your glow up by completing this weekly check-in. You'll plan ahead and set the tone for the week while reminding yourself of your glowed up goals!

ROUTINES AND SCHEDULE

I'm going to commit to these goals:

○ _____
○ _____
○ _____
○ _____

I'm working on these healthy habits:

○ _____
○ _____
○ _____
○ _____

I'm going to stay on track by:

○ _____
○ _____
○ _____
○ _____

DIET AND EXERCISE

Healthy foods I'm eating more of:

○ _____
○ _____
○ _____
○ _____

This week's superstar supplement(s):

○ _____
○ _____
○ _____
○ _____

This week's movement goals:

○ _____
○ _____
○ _____
○ _____

BEAUTY AND STYLE

I will look and feel my best by:

○ _____
○ _____
○ _____
○ _____

I will add glamour to my routine by:

○ _____
○ _____
○ _____
○ _____

I will pamper myself by:

○ _____
○ _____
○ _____
○ _____

My big glow up goal for the year is:

This week, I will get closer to my glow up goal by:

I affirm that I *am*:

This week's self-care activities for my:

Mind	Body	Soul
M	M	M
T	T	T
W	W	W
T	T	T
F	F	F
S	S	S
S	S	S

Daily
CHECK-IN

At the end of each day, use the following prompts to check in with yourself and your glow up progress, filling in the chart with your reflections.

MONDAY	TUESDAY	WEDNESDAY

I'm grateful for this:

Glow up wins from today:

Things to remember for tomorrow:

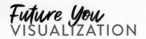

Future You
VISUALIZATION

Now, use your vision board to visualize about your glowed up future for five minutes. Trust that you are becoming your best and baddest self. Your glow up is under way—keep going!

THURSDAY	FRIDAY	SATURDAY	SUNDAY

Sunday
CHECK-IN

Every Sunday, create dedicated Me Time for you and your glow up by completing this weekly check-in. You'll plan ahead and set the tone for the week while reminding yourself of your glowed up goals!

ROUTINES AND SCHEDULE

I'm going to commit to these goals:

○ _____
○ _____
○ _____
○ _____

I'm working on these healthy habits:

○ _____
○ _____
○ _____
○ _____

I'm going to stay on track by:

○ _____
○ _____
○ _____
○ _____

DIET AND EXERCISE

Healthy foods I'm eating more of:

○ _____
○ _____
○ _____
○ _____

This week's superstar supplement(s):

○ _____
○ _____
○ _____
○ _____

This week's movement goals:

○ _____
○ _____
○ _____
○ _____

BEAUTY AND STYLE

I will look and feel my best by:

○ _____
○ _____
○ _____
○ _____

I will add glamour to my routine by:

○ _____
○ _____
○ _____
○ _____

I will pamper myself by:

○ _____
○ _____
○ _____
○ _____

My big glow up goal for the year is:

This week, I will get closer to my glow up goal by:

I affirm that I *am*:

This week's self-care activities for my:

Mind	Body	Soul
M	M	M
T	T	T
W	W	W
T	T	T
F	F	F
S	S	S
S	S	S

Daily
CHECK-IN

At the end of each day, use the following prompts to check in with yourself and your glow up progress, filling in the chart with your reflections.

MONDAY	TUESDAY	WEDNESDAY

I'm grateful for this:

Glow up wins from today:

Things to remember for tomorrow:

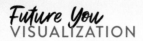

Future You
VISUALIZATION

Now, use your vision board to visualize about your glowed up future for five minutes. Trust that you are becoming your best and baddest self. Your glow up is under way—keep going!

THURSDAY	FRIDAY	SATURDAY	SUNDAY

Sunday
CHECK-IN

Every Sunday, create dedicated Me Time for you and your glow up by completing this weekly check-in. You'll plan ahead and set the tone for the week while reminding yourself of your glowed up goals!

ROUTINES AND SCHEDULE

I'm going to commit to these goals:

○ _____
○ _____
○ _____
○ _____

I'm working on these healthy habits:

○ _____
○ _____
○ _____
○ _____

I'm going to stay on track by:

○ _____
○ _____
○ _____
○ _____

DIET AND EXERCISE

Healthy foods I'm eating more of:

○ _____
○ _____
○ _____
○ _____

This week's superstar supplement(s):

○ _____
○ _____
○ _____
○ _____

This week's movement goals:

○ _____
○ _____
○ _____
○ _____

BEAUTY AND STYLE

I will look and feel my best by:

○ _____
○ _____
○ _____
○ _____

I will add glamour to my routine by:

○ _____
○ _____
○ _____
○ _____

I will pamper myself by:

○ _____
○ _____
○ _____
○ _____

My big glow up goal for the year is:

This week, I will get closer to my glow up goal by:

I affirm that I *am*:

This week's self-care activities for my:

Mind	Body	Soul
M	M	M
T	T	T
W	W	W
T	T	T
F	F	F
S	S	S
S	S	S

Daily
CHECK-IN

At the end of each day, use the following prompts to check in with yourself and your glow up progress, filling in the chart with your reflections.

MONDAY	TUESDAY	WEDNESDAY

I'm grateful for this:

Glow up wins from today:

Things to remember for tomorrow:

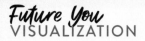

Future You
VISUALIZATION

Now, use your vision board to visualize about your glowed up future for five minutes. Trust that you are becoming your best and baddest self. Your glow up is under way—keep going!

THURSDAY	FRIDAY	SATURDAY	SUNDAY

Sunday
CHECK-IN

Every Sunday, create dedicated Me Time for you and your glow up by completing this weekly check-in. You'll plan ahead and set the tone for the week while reminding yourself of your glowed up goals!

ROUTINES AND SCHEDULE

I'm going to commit to these goals:

○ _____
○ _____
○ _____
○ _____

I'm working on these healthy habits:

○ _____
○ _____
○ _____
○ _____

I'm going to stay on track by:

○ _____
○ _____
○ _____
○ _____

DIET AND EXERCISE

Healthy foods I'm eating more of:

○ _____
○ _____
○ _____
○ _____

This week's superstar supplement(s):

○ _____
○ _____
○ _____
○ _____

This week's movement goals:

○ _____
○ _____
○ _____
○ _____

BEAUTY AND STYLE

I will look and feel my best by:

○ _____
○ _____
○ _____
○ _____

I will add glamour to my routine by:

○ _____
○ _____
○ _____
○ _____

I will pamper myself by:

○ _____
○ _____
○ _____
○ _____

My big glow up goal for the year is:

This week, I will get closer to my glow up goal by:

I affirm that I *am*:

HOLISTIC TOOLS AND PRACTICES FOR WELLNESS

This week's self-care activities for my:

Mind	Body	Soul
M	M	M
T	T	T
W	W	W
T	T	T
F	F	F
S	S	S
S	S	S

Daily
CHECK-IN

At the end of each day, use the following prompts to check in with yourself and your glow up progress, filling in the chart with your reflections.

MONDAY	TUESDAY	WEDNESDAY

I'm grateful for this:

Glow up wins from today:

Things to remember for tomorrow:

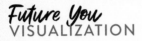 Future You
VISUALIZATION

Now, use your vision board to visualize about your glowed up future for five minutes. Trust that you are becoming your best and baddest self. Your glow up is under way—keep going!

THURSDAY	FRIDAY	SATURDAY	SUNDAY

Sunday
CHECK-IN

Every Sunday, create dedicated Me Time for you and your glow up by completing this weekly check-in. You'll plan ahead and set the tone for the week while reminding yourself of your glowed up goals!

ROUTINES AND SCHEDULE

I'm going to commit to these goals:

- ○ _____
- ○ _____
- ○ _____
- ○ _____

I'm working on these healthy habits:

- ○ _____
- ○ _____
- ○ _____
- ○ _____

I'm going to stay on track by:

- ○ _____
- ○ _____
- ○ _____
- ○ _____

DIET AND EXERCISE

Healthy foods I'm eating more of:

- ○ _____
- ○ _____
- ○ _____
- ○ _____

This week's superstar supplement(s):

- ○ _____
- ○ _____
- ○ _____
- ○ _____

This week's movement goals:

- ○ _____
- ○ _____
- ○ _____
- ○ _____

BEAUTY AND STYLE

I will look and feel my best by:

- ○ _____
- ○ _____
- ○ _____
- ○ _____

I will add glamour to my routine by:

- ○ _____
- ○ _____
- ○ _____
- ○ _____

I will pamper myself by:

- ○ _____
- ○ _____
- ○ _____
- ○ _____

My big glow up goal for the year is:

This week, I will get closer to my glow up goal by:

I affirm that I *am*:

This week's self-care activities for my:

Mind	Body	Soul
M	M	M
T	T	T
W	W	W
T	T	T
F	F	F
S	S	S
S	S	S

Daily
CHECK-IN

At the end of each day, use the following prompts to check in with yourself and your glow up progress, filling in the chart with your reflections.

MONDAY	TUESDAY	WEDNESDAY

I'm grateful for this:

Glow up wins from today:

Things to remember for tomorrow:

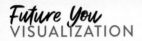

Future You
VISUALIZATION

Now, use your vision board to visualize about your glowed up future for five minutes. Trust that you are becoming your best and baddest self. Your glow up is under way—keep going!

THURSDAY	FRIDAY	SATURDAY	SUNDAY

Sunday
CHECK-IN

Every Sunday, create dedicated Me Time for you and your glow up by completing this weekly check-in. You'll plan ahead and set the tone for the week while reminding yourself of your glowed up goals!

ROUTINES AND SCHEDULE

I'm going to commit to these goals:

- ○ _____
- ○ _____
- ○ _____
- ○ _____

I'm working on these healthy habits:

- ○ _____
- ○ _____
- ○ _____
- ○ _____

I'm going to stay on track by:

- ○ _____
- ○ _____
- ○ _____
- ○ _____

DIET AND EXERCISE

Healthy foods I'm eating more of:

- ○ _____
- ○ _____
- ○ _____
- ○ _____

This week's superstar supplement(s):

- ○ _____
- ○ _____
- ○ _____
- ○ _____

This week's movement goals:

- ○ _____
- ○ _____
- ○ _____
- ○ _____

BEAUTY AND STYLE

I will look and feel my best by:

- ○ _____
- ○ _____
- ○ _____
- ○ _____

I will add glamour to my routine by:

- ○ _____
- ○ _____
- ○ _____
- ○ _____

I will pamper myself by:

- ○ _____
- ○ _____
- ○ _____
- ○ _____

My big glow up goal for the year is:

This week, I will get closer to my glow up goal by:

I affirm that I *am*:

This week's self-care activities for my:

Mind	Body	Soul
M	M	M
T	T	T
W	W	W
T	T	T
F	F	F
S	S	S
S	S	S

Daily
CHECK-IN

At the end of each day, use the following prompts to check in with yourself and your glow up progress, filling in the chart with your reflections.

MONDAY	TUESDAY	WEDNESDAY

I'm grateful for this:

Glow up wins from today:

Things to remember for tomorrow:

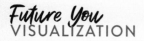

Future You
VISUALIZATION

Now, use your vision board to visualize about your glowed up future for five minutes. Trust that you are becoming your best and baddest self. Your glow up is under way—keep going!

THURSDAY	FRIDAY	SATURDAY	SUNDAY

Sunday
CHECK-IN

Every Sunday, create dedicated Me Time for you and your glow up by completing this weekly check-in. You'll plan ahead and set the tone for the week while reminding yourself of your glowed up goals!

ROUTINES AND SCHEDULE

I'm going to commit to these goals:

○ _____
○ _____
○ _____
○ _____

I'm working on these healthy habits:

○ _____
○ _____
○ _____
○ _____

I'm going to stay on track by:

○ _____
○ _____
○ _____
○ _____

DIET AND EXERCISE

Healthy foods I'm eating more of:

○ _____
○ _____
○ _____
○ _____

This week's superstar supplement(s):

○ _____
○ _____
○ _____
○ _____

This week's movement goals:

○ _____
○ _____
○ _____
○ _____

BEAUTY AND STYLE

I will look and feel my best by:

○ _____
○ _____
○ _____
○ _____

I will add glamour to my routine by:

○ _____
○ _____
○ _____
○ _____

I will pamper myself by:

○ _____
○ _____
○ _____
○ _____

VISUALIZING AND PREPARING FOR YOUR DREAM LIFE

My big glow up goal for the year is:

This week, I will get closer to my glow up goal by:

I affirm that I *am*:

HOLISTIC TOOLS AND PRACTICES FOR WELLNESS

This week's self-care activities for my:

Mind	Body	Soul
M	M	M
T	T	T
W	W	W
T	T	T
F	F	F
S	S	S
S	S	S

Daily
CHECK-IN

At the end of each day, use the following prompts to check in with yourself and your glow up progress, filling in the chart with your reflections.

MONDAY	TUESDAY	WEDNESDAY

I'm grateful for this:

Glow up wins from today:

Things to remember for tomorrow:

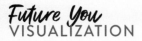
Future You
VISUALIZATION

Now, use your vision board to visualize about your glowed up future for five minutes. Trust that you are becoming your best and baddest self. Your glow up is under way—keep going!

THURSDAY	FRIDAY	SATURDAY	SUNDAY

Sunday
CHECK-IN

Every Sunday, create dedicated Me Time for you and your glow up by completing this weekly check-in. You'll plan ahead and set the tone for the week while reminding yourself of your glowed up goals!

ROUTINES AND SCHEDULE

I'm going to commit to these goals:

- ○ ....
- ○ ....
- ○ ....
- ○ ....

I'm working on these healthy habits:

- ○ ....
- ○ ....
- ○ ....
- ○ ....

I'm going to stay on track by:

- ○ ....
- ○ ....
- ○ ....
- ○ ....

DIET AND EXERCISE

Healthy foods I'm eating more of:

- ○ ....
- ○ ....
- ○ ....
- ○ ....

This week's superstar supplement(s):

- ○ ....
- ○ ....
- ○ ....
- ○ ....

This week's movement goals:

- ○ ....
- ○ ....
- ○ ....
- ○ ....

BEAUTY AND STYLE

I will look and feel my best by:

- ○ ....
- ○ ....
- ○ ....
- ○ ....

I will add glamour to my routine by:

- ○ ....
- ○ ....
- ○ ....
- ○ ....

I will pamper myself by:

- ○ ....
- ○ ....
- ○ ....
- ○ ....

My big glow up goal for the year is:

This week, I will get closer to my glow up goal by:

I affirm that I *am*:

This week's self-care activities for my:

Mind	Body	Soul
M	M	M
T	T	T
W	W	W
T	T	T
F	F	F
S	S	S
S	S	S

Daily
CHECK-IN

At the end of each day, use the following prompts to check in with yourself and your glow up progress, filling in the chart with your reflections.

MONDAY	TUESDAY	WEDNESDAY

I'm grateful for this:

Glow up wins from today:

Things to remember for tomorrow:

Future You
VISUALIZATION

Now, use your vision board to visualize about your glowed up future for five minutes. Trust that you are becoming your best and baddest self. Your glow up is under way—keep going!

THURSDAY	FRIDAY	SATURDAY	SUNDAY

Sunday
CHECK-IN

Every Sunday, create dedicated Me Time for you and your glow up by completing this weekly check-in. You'll plan ahead and set the tone for the week while reminding yourself of your glowed up goals!

ROUTINES AND SCHEDULE

I'm going to commit to these goals:

○ _____
○ _____
○ _____
○ _____

I'm working on these healthy habits:

○ _____
○ _____
○ _____
○ _____

I'm going to stay on track by:

○ _____
○ _____
○ _____
○ _____

DIET AND EXERCISE

Healthy foods I'm eating more of:

○ _____
○ _____
○ _____
○ _____

This week's superstar supplement(s):

○ _____
○ _____
○ _____
○ _____

This week's movement goals:

○ _____
○ _____
○ _____
○ _____

BEAUTY AND STYLE

I will look and feel my best by:

○ _____
○ _____
○ _____
○ _____

I will add glamour to my routine by:

○ _____
○ _____
○ _____
○ _____

I will pamper myself by:

○ _____
○ _____
○ _____
○ _____

VISUALIZING AND PREPARING FOR YOUR DREAM LIFE

My big glow up goal for the year is:

This week, I will get closer to my glow up goal by:

I affirm that I *am*:

HOLISTIC TOOLS AND PRACTICES FOR WELLNESS

This week's self-care activities for my:

Mind	Body	Soul
M	M	M
T	T	T
W	W	W
T	T	T
F	F	F
S	S	S
S	S	S

Daily
CHECK-IN

At the end of each day, use the following prompts to check in with yourself and your glow up progress, filling in the chart with your reflections.

	MONDAY	TUESDAY	WEDNESDAY
I'm grateful for this:			
Glow up wins from today:			
Things to remember for tomorrow:			

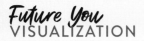

VISUALIZATION

Now, use your vision board to visualize about your glowed up future for five minutes. Trust that you are becoming your best and baddest self. Your glow up is under way—keep going!

THURSDAY	FRIDAY	SATURDAY	SUNDAY

Sunday
CHECK-IN

Every Sunday, create dedicated Me Time for you and your glow up by completing this weekly check-in. You'll plan ahead and set the tone for the week while reminding yourself of your glowed up goals!

ROUTINES AND SCHEDULE

I'm going to commit to these goals:

○ _____
○ _____
○ _____
○ _____

I'm working on these healthy habits:

○ _____
○ _____
○ _____
○ _____

I'm going to stay on track by:

○ _____
○ _____
○ _____
○ _____

DIET AND EXERCISE

Healthy foods I'm eating more of:

○ _____
○ _____
○ _____
○ _____

This week's superstar supplement(s):

○ _____
○ _____
○ _____
○ _____

This week's movement goals:

○ _____
○ _____
○ _____
○ _____

BEAUTY AND STYLE

I will look and feel my best by:

○ _____
○ _____
○ _____
○ _____

I will add glamour to my routine by:

○ _____
○ _____
○ _____
○ _____

I will pamper myself by:

○ _____
○ _____
○ _____
○ _____

VISUALIZING AND PREPARING FOR YOUR DREAM LIFE

My big glow up goal for the year is:

This week, I will get closer to my glow up goal by:

I affirm that I *am*:

HOLISTIC TOOLS AND PRACTICES FOR WELLNESS

This week's self-care activities for my:

Mind	Body	Soul
M	M	M
T	T	T
W	W	W
T	T	T
F	F	F
S	S	S
S	S	S

Daily
CHECK-IN

At the end of each day, use the following prompts to check in with yourself and your glow up progress, filling in the chart with your reflections.

MONDAY	TUESDAY	WEDNESDAY

I'm grateful for this:

Glow up wins from today:

Things to remember for tomorrow:

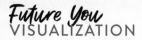
VISUALIZATION

Now, use your vision board to visualize about your glowed up future for five minutes. Trust that you are becoming your best and baddest self. Your glow up is under way—keep going!

THURSDAY	FRIDAY	SATURDAY	SUNDAY

Sunday
CHECK-IN

Every Sunday, create dedicated Me Time for you and your glow up by completing this weekly check-in. You'll plan ahead and set the tone for the week while reminding yourself of your glowed up goals!

ROUTINES AND SCHEDULE

I'm going to commit to these goals:

- ○ _____
- ○ _____
- ○ _____
- ○ _____

I'm working on these healthy habits:

- ○ _____
- ○ _____
- ○ _____
- ○ _____

I'm going to stay on track by:

- ○ _____
- ○ _____
- ○ _____
- ○ _____

DIET AND EXERCISE

Healthy foods I'm eating more of:

- ○ _____
- ○ _____
- ○ _____
- ○ _____

This week's superstar supplement(s):

- ○ _____
- ○ _____
- ○ _____
- ○ _____

This week's movement goals:

- ○ _____
- ○ _____
- ○ _____
- ○ _____

BEAUTY AND STYLE

I will look and feel my best by:

- ○ _____
- ○ _____
- ○ _____
- ○ _____

I will add glamour to my routine by:

- ○ _____
- ○ _____
- ○ _____
- ○ _____

I will pamper myself by:

- ○ _____
- ○ _____
- ○ _____
- ○ _____

VISUALIZING AND PREPARING FOR YOUR DREAM LIFE

My big glow up goal for the year is:

This week, I will get closer to my glow up goal by:

I affirm that I *am*:

HOLISTIC TOOLS AND PRACTICES FOR WELLNESS

This week's self-care activities for my:

Mind	Body	Soul
M	M	M
T	T	T
W	W	W
T	T	T
F	F	F
S	S	S
S	S	S

Daily
CHECK-IN

At the end of each day, use the following prompts to check in with yourself and your glow up progress, filling in the chart with your reflections.

MONDAY	TUESDAY	WEDNESDAY

I'm grateful for this:

Glow up wins from today:

Things to remember for tomorrow:

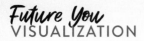

Future You
VISUALIZATION

Now, use your vision board to visualize about your glowed up future for five minutes. Trust that you are becoming your best and baddest self. Your glow up is under way—keep going!

THURSDAY	FRIDAY	SATURDAY	SUNDAY

Sunday
CHECK-IN

Every Sunday, create dedicated Me Time for you and your glow up by completing this weekly check-in. You'll plan ahead and set the tone for the week while reminding yourself of your glowed up goals!

ROUTINES AND SCHEDULE

I'm going to commit to these goals:

○ _____
○ _____
○ _____
○ _____

I'm working on these healthy habits:

○ _____
○ _____
○ _____
○ _____

I'm going to stay on track by:

○ _____
○ _____
○ _____
○ _____

DIET AND EXERCISE

Healthy foods I'm eating more of:

○ _____
○ _____
○ _____
○ _____

This week's superstar supplement(s):

○ _____
○ _____
○ _____
○ _____

This week's movement goals:

○ _____
○ _____
○ _____
○ _____

BEAUTY AND STYLE

I will look and feel my best by:

○ _____
○ _____
○ _____
○ _____

I will add glamour to my routine by:

○ _____
○ _____
○ _____
○ _____

I will pamper myself by:

○ _____
○ _____
○ _____
○ _____

My big glow up goal for the year is:

This week, I will get closer to my glow up goal by:

I affirm that I *am*:

HOLISTIC TOOLS AND PRACTICES FOR WELLNESS

This week's self-care activities for my:

Mind	Body	Soul
M	M	M
T	T	T
W	W	W
T	T	T
F	F	F
S	S	S
S	S	S

Daily
CHECK-IN

At the end of each day, use the following prompts to check in with yourself and your glow up progress, filling in the chart with your reflections.

MONDAY	TUESDAY	WEDNESDAY

I'm grateful for this:

Glow up wins from today:

Things to remember for tomorrow:

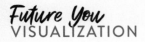
Future You
VISUALIZATION

Now, use your vision board to visualize about your glowed up future for five minutes. Trust that you are becoming your best and baddest self. Your glow up is under way—keep going!

THURSDAY	FRIDAY	SATURDAY	SUNDAY

Sunday
CHECK-IN

Every Sunday, create dedicated Me Time for you and your glow up by completing this weekly check-in. You'll plan ahead and set the tone for the week while reminding yourself of your glowed up goals!

ROUTINES AND SCHEDULE

I'm going to commit to these goals:

○ _____
○ _____
○ _____
○ _____

I'm working on these healthy habits:

○ _____
○ _____
○ _____
○ _____

I'm going to stay on track by:

○ _____
○ _____
○ _____
○ _____

DIET AND EXERCISE

Healthy foods I'm eating more of:

○ _____
○ _____
○ _____
○ _____

This week's superstar supplement(s):

○ _____
○ _____
○ _____
○ _____

This week's movement goals:

○ _____
○ _____
○ _____
○ _____

BEAUTY AND STYLE

I will look and feel my best by:

○ _____
○ _____
○ _____
○ _____

I will add glamour to my routine by:

○ _____
○ _____
○ _____
○ _____

I will pamper myself by:

○ _____
○ _____
○ _____
○ _____

My big glow up goal for the year is:

This week, I will get closer to my glow up goal by:

I affirm that I *am*:

This week's self-care activities for my:

Mind	**Body**	**Soul**
M	M	M
T	T	T
W	W	W
T	T	T
F	F	F
S	S	S
S	S	S

Daily
CHECK-IN

At the end of each day, use the following prompts to check in with yourself and your glow up progress, filling in the chart with your reflections.

MONDAY	TUESDAY	WEDNESDAY

I'm grateful for this:

Glow up wins from today:

Things to remember for tomorrow:

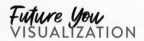
Future You
VISUALIZATION

Now, use your vision board to visualize about your glowed up future for five minutes. Trust that you are becoming your best and baddest self. Your glow up is under way—keep going!

THURSDAY	FRIDAY	SATURDAY	SUNDAY

Sunday
CHECK-IN

Every Sunday, create dedicated Me Time for you and your glow up by completing this weekly check-in. You'll plan ahead and set the tone for the week while reminding yourself of your glowed up goals!

ROUTINES AND SCHEDULE

I'm going to commit to these goals:

- ○ _____
- ○ _____
- ○ _____
- ○ _____

I'm working on these healthy habits:

- ○ _____
- ○ _____
- ○ _____
- ○ _____

I'm going to stay on track by:

- ○ _____
- ○ _____
- ○ _____
- ○ _____

DIET AND EXERCISE

Healthy foods I'm eating more of:

- ○ _____
- ○ _____
- ○ _____
- ○ _____

This week's superstar supplement(s):

- ○ _____
- ○ _____
- ○ _____
- ○ _____

This week's movement goals:

- ○ _____
- ○ _____
- ○ _____
- ○ _____

BEAUTY AND STYLE

I will look and feel my best by:

- ○ _____
- ○ _____
- ○ _____
- ○ _____

I will add glamour to my routine by:

- ○ _____
- ○ _____
- ○ _____
- ○ _____

I will pamper myself by:

- ○ _____
- ○ _____
- ○ _____
- ○ _____

VISUALIZING AND PREPARING FOR YOUR DREAM LIFE

My big glow up goal for the year is:

This week, I will get closer to my glow up goal by:

I affirm that I *am*:

HOLISTIC TOOLS AND PRACTICES FOR WELLNESS

This week's self-care activities for my:

Mind	Body	Soul
M	M	M
T	T	T
W	W	W
T	T	T
F	F	F
S	S	S
S	S	S

Daily
CHECK-IN

At the end of each day, use the following prompts to check in with yourself and your glow up progress, filling in the chart with your reflections.

MONDAY	TUESDAY	WEDNESDAY

I'm grateful for this:

Glow up wins from today:

Things to remember for tomorrow:

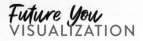
Future You
VISUALIZATION

Now, use your vision board to visualize about your glowed up future for five minutes. Trust that you are becoming your best and baddest self. Your glow up is under way—keep going!

THURSDAY	FRIDAY	SATURDAY	SUNDAY

Sunday CHECK-IN

Every Sunday, create dedicated Me Time for you and your glow up by completing this weekly check-in. You'll plan ahead and set the tone for the week while reminding yourself of your glowed up goals!

ROUTINES AND SCHEDULE

I'm going to commit to these goals:

- ○ _____
- ○ _____
- ○ _____
- ○ _____

I'm working on these healthy habits:

- ○ _____
- ○ _____
- ○ _____
- ○ _____

I'm going to stay on track by:

- ○ _____
- ○ _____
- ○ _____
- ○ _____

DIET AND EXERCISE

Healthy foods I'm eating more of:

- ○ _____
- ○ _____
- ○ _____
- ○ _____

This week's superstar supplement(s):

- ○ _____
- ○ _____
- ○ _____
- ○ _____

This week's movement goals:

- ○ _____
- ○ _____
- ○ _____
- ○ _____

BEAUTY AND STYLE

I will look and feel my best by:

- ○ _____
- ○ _____
- ○ _____
- ○ _____

I will add glamour to my routine by:

- ○ _____
- ○ _____
- ○ _____
- ○ _____

I will pamper myself by:

- ○ _____
- ○ _____
- ○ _____
- ○ _____

My big glow up goal for the year is:

This week, I will get closer to my glow up goal by:

I affirm that I *am*:

This week's self-care activities for my:

Mind	Body	Soul
M	M	M
T	T	T
W	W	W
T	T	T
F	F	F
S	S	S
S	S	S

Daily
CHECK-IN

At the end of each day, use the following prompts to check in with yourself and your glow up progress, filling in the chart with your reflections.

	MONDAY	TUESDAY	WEDNESDAY
I'm grateful for this:			
Glow up wins from today:			
Things to remember for tomorrow:			

Future You
VISUALIZATION

Now, use your vision board to visualize about your glowed up future for five minutes. Trust that you are becoming your best and baddest self. Your glow up is under way—keep going!

THURSDAY	FRIDAY	SATURDAY	SUNDAY

Sunday
CHECK-IN

Every Sunday, create dedicated Me Time for you and your glow up by completing this weekly check-in. You'll plan ahead and set the tone for the week while reminding yourself of your glowed up goals!

ROUTINES AND SCHEDULE

I'm going to commit to these goals:

○ _____
○ _____
○ _____
○ _____

I'm working on these healthy habits:

○ _____
○ _____
○ _____
○ _____

I'm going to stay on track by:

○ _____
○ _____
○ _____
○ _____

DIET AND EXERCISE

Healthy foods I'm eating more of:

○ _____
○ _____
○ _____
○ _____

This week's superstar supplement(s):

○ _____
○ _____
○ _____
○ _____

This week's movement goals:

○ _____
○ _____
○ _____
○ _____

BEAUTY AND STYLE

I will look and feel my best by:

○ _____
○ _____
○ _____
○ _____

I will add glamour to my routine by:

○ _____
○ _____
○ _____
○ _____

I will pamper myself by:

○ _____
○ _____
○ _____
○ _____

VISUALIZING AND PREPARING FOR YOUR DREAM LIFE

My big glow up goal for the year is:

This week, I will get closer to my glow up goal by:

I affirm that I *am*:

HOLISTIC TOOLS AND PRACTICES FOR WELLNESS

This week's self-care activities for my:

Mind	Body	Soul
M	M	M
T	T	T
W	W	W
T	T	T
F	F	F
S	S	S
S	S	S

Daily
CHECK-IN

At the end of each day, use the following prompts to check in with yourself and your glow up progress, filling in the chart with your reflections.

MONDAY	TUESDAY	WEDNESDAY

I'm grateful for this:

Glow up wins from today:

Things to remember for tomorrow:

Future You
VISUALIZATION

Now, use your vision board to visualize about your glowed up future for five minutes. Trust that you are becoming your best and baddest self. Your glow up is under way—keep going!

THURSDAY	FRIDAY	SATURDAY	SUNDAY

Sunday
CHECK-IN

Every Sunday, create dedicated Me Time for you and your glow up by completing this weekly check-in. You'll plan ahead and set the tone for the week while reminding yourself of your glowed up goals!

ROUTINES AND SCHEDULE

I'm going to commit to these goals:

○ _____
○ _____
○ _____
○ _____

I'm working on these healthy habits:

○ _____
○ _____
○ _____
○ _____

I'm going to stay on track by:

○ _____
○ _____
○ _____
○ _____

DIET AND EXERCISE

Healthy foods I'm eating more of:

○ _____
○ _____
○ _____
○ _____

This week's superstar supplement(s):

○ _____
○ _____
○ _____
○ _____

This week's movement goals:

○ _____
○ _____
○ _____
○ _____

BEAUTY AND STYLE

I will look and feel my best by:

○ _____
○ _____
○ _____
○ _____

I will add glamour to my routine by:

○ _____
○ _____
○ _____
○ _____

I will pamper myself by:

○ _____
○ _____
○ _____
○ _____

My big glow up goal for the year is:

This week, I will get closer to my glow up goal by:

I affirm that I *am*:

HOLISTIC TOOLS AND PRACTICES FOR WELLNESS

This week's self-care activities for my:

Mind	Body	Soul
M	M	M
T	T	T
W	W	W
T	T	T
F	F	F
S	S	S
S	S	S

Daily
CHECK-IN

At the end of each day, use the following prompts to check in with yourself and your glow up progress, filling in the chart with your reflections.

	MONDAY	TUESDAY	WEDNESDAY
I'm grateful for this:			
Glow up wins from today:			
Things to remember for tomorrow:			

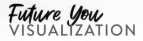
Future You
VISUALIZATION

Now, use your vision board to visualize about your glowed up future for five minutes. Trust that you are becoming your best and baddest self. Your glow up is under way—keep going!

THURSDAY	FRIDAY	SATURDAY	SUNDAY

About the Author

Dr. Danielle Richardson is a Los Angeles–based optometrist, yoga teacher, and wellness entrepreneur. She is the founder of Fierce Clarity, a holistic wellness and lifestyle space for modern professionals. She takes a holistic approach to wellness in her own life and is passionate about sharing these tools and practices with others. Dr. Danielle's science background and yogic studies blend together to create her unique approach to total well-being of the mind, body, and soul. She focuses on creating evidence-based wellness content to empower busy people to make healthier decisions. She has hosted international yoga retreats, corporate wellness programming, and pop-up events that introduce mindful and health-conscious living to a modern audience.